Critical Care

of related interest

Spiritual Care in Practice
Case Studies in Healthcare Chaplaincy
Edited by George Fitchett and Steve Nolan
Foreword by Christina Puchalski
Afterword by John Swinton
ISBN 978 1 84905 976 3
eISBN 978 0 85700 876 3

Multifaith Care for Sick and Dying
Children and their Families
A Multi-disciplinary Guide
Paul Nash, Madeleine Parkes and Zamir Hussain
ISBN 978 1 84905 606 9
eISBN 978 1 78450 072 6

Spiritual Care at the End of Life
The Chaplain as a 'Hopeful Presence'
Steve Nolan
ISBN 978 1 84905 199 6
eISBN 978 0 85700 513 7

Making Sense of Spirituality in Nursing
and Health Care Practice
An Interactive Approach
Second Edition
Wilfred McSherry
Foreword by Keith Cash
ISBN 978 1 84310 365 3
eISBN 978 1 84642 530 1

Critical Care

Delivering Spiritual Care
in Healthcare Contexts

Edited by
Jonathan Pye, Peter Sedgwick
and Andrew Todd

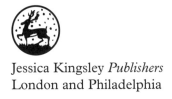

Jessica Kingsley *Publishers*
London and Philadelphia

List on pp.111–12 reproduced under the terms of the Open Government Licence v 3.0.
List on p.27 reproduced with kind permission of the Royal College of Nursing.

First published in 2015
by Jessica Kingsley Publishers
73 Collier Street
London N1 9BE, UK
and
400 Market Street, Suite 400
Philadelphia, PA 19106, USA

www.jkp.com

Library of Congress Cataloging in Publication Data
Critical care (Pye)
   Critical care : delivering spiritual care in healthcare contexts
/ edited by Jonathan Pye, Peter Sedgwick
and Andrew Todd.
      p. ; cm.
   Includes bibliographical references and index.
   ISBN 978-1-84905-497-3 (alk. paper)
   I. Pye, Jonathan H., editor. II. Sedgwick, P. H. (Peter
Humphrey), 1948- , editor. III. Todd, Andrew, 1961-
, editor. IV. Title.
   [DNLM: 1. Pastoral Care. 2. Critical Care. 3. Spirituality. WM 61]
   R726.8
   616.02'8--dc23
                              2015003712

British Library Cataloguing in Publication Data
A CIP catalogue record for this book is available from the British Library

ISBN 978 1 84905 497 3
eISBN 978 0 85700 901 2

Printed and bound in Great Britain

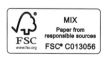

CONTENTS

PREFACE

There are few today who would argue that contemporary healthcare is not in a state of crisis. In increasingly market-driven contexts, where the focus is all too often on outcomes and targets, the danger is that the focus of healthcare has systematically shifted away from the person and onto the healthcare systems themselves. This, of course, is not to argue that politics and economics do not have their part to play – of course they do, but especially in the high-tech world of Western medicine and healthcare so do other perspectives, including those of anthropology, sociology, philosophy, law and, not least, theology whose voices have in the past too often been disregarded, but whose practitioners, and theorists, are the co-workers of doctors, nurses and those in other allied professions, and who have much to contribute from their own distinctive perspectives.

This book is the result of a collaboration between academics and practitioners, each of whom has a professional interest in healthcare, and in spiritual care in particular. Its premise is that academic research and healthcare practice need each other – research needs to be grounded in practice, practice needs to be informed by research. Whilst this book is primarily one that is about spiritual care, at a time when it is being increasingly recognised that good healthcare – a healthcare that focuses on the needs and well-being of care-receivers – is best practised in interdisciplinary ways, it also argues that the lessons learned from rigorous research into, and reflection on the practice of spiritual care can inform the research and practice of other disciplines, including those for whom 'spiritual' care may have in the past seemed an odd bedfellow. In this project, then, the starting point is the patient as person, viewed holistically, and the premise that such person-centred care necessarily involves that which transcends the physical alone.

The contributions in this volume are diverse and represent a broad spectrum of methodologies and of healthcare contexts. They recognise the changing context of healthcare in a plural world and are committed to healthcare as a common enterprise. Although the proximate context of what has been written is the UK National Health Service, the insights and observations contained within this book are applicable to other healthcare systems, too. What it offers then, is not answers but a contribution to the debate and an openness to a continuing dialogue.

Jonathan H. Pye
Editor

PART 1

Constructing Spiritual Care

CHAPTER 1

The Narrative of Spiritual Care

Locating Models of Spiritual Care within
Contemporary Healthcare Education and Practice

Jonathan H. Pye

Why is it that I owe something more to my physician and my teacher, and yet do not complete the payment of what is due to them? It is because from being physician and teacher they become friends, and we are under an obligation to them, not because of their skill, which they sell, but because of their kind and friendly goodwill.

If, therefore, a physician does no more than feel my pulse and put me on the list of those whom he visits on his rounds, instructing me what to do and what to avoid without any personal feeling, I owe him nothing more than his fee, since he sees me not so much as a friend, as one who summons him.[1] Why, then, are we so much indebted to these men? Not because what they have sold us is worth more than we have paid for it, but because they have contributed something to us personally. A physician who gave me more attention than was necessary, because he was concerned for me, not for his professional reputation; who was not content to prescribe remedies, but also applied them; who sat at my bedside among my anxious friends and hurried to me at times of crisis; for whom no service was too burdensome, none too distasteful to perform; one who was not indifferent to my moans; to whom, although a host of others sent for him, I was always his chief concern... Such a man has placed me under an obligation not so much as a physician as a friend. (Seneca, De Beneficiis, Book IV section 16)

The Stoic philosopher, Seneca writing in the 1st century CE, asks the question that lies both at the heart of this chapter and of contemporary healthcare's search to discover why, despite all the advances in contemporary medical technology, people often remain so dissatisfied with the treatment they receive from their doctors and other healthcare professionals in increasingly target-driven and cost-orientated health-care systems. At the heart of this dissatisfaction is the feeling that they are increasingly being regarded as simply another medical statistic, the object of care, rather than its subject and that they are no longer regarded as a 'person' with their own unique history but as a 'case', a 'problem' to be solved or, worse still, a medical 'failure' to be moved on from when cure is no longer an option.

Harvey Chochinov (2007), writing in the *British Medical Journal* about human dignity and the essence of medicine, begins with a quote from the late American essayist, Anatole Broyard (1992), who was facing a terminal metastatic prostate cancer, with words redolent of those of Seneca 2000 years earlier:

> *To the typical physician my illness is a routine incident in his rounds while for me it's the crisis of my life. I would feel better if I had a doctor who at least perceived this incongruity... I just wish he would...give me his whole mind just once, be bonded with me for a brief space survey my soul as well as my flesh, to get at my illness, for each man is ill in his own way. (Chochinov 2007, p.184)*

Despite the plea for such patient individuality, many of those engaged in the practice of medicine and healthcare today complain that they simply do not have the time to listen to patients or share their stories. Some suggest that even the attentive art of taking a full patient history is a skill that has been sadly neglected, maybe even lost, in the technological busyness of contemporary medical education and practice.

Although this lack of engagement is often regarded as a *sequela* of contemporary trends in healthcare, at least in Western industrialised societies, this displacement of the 'person' in the modern period is something that has been going on since at least the time of the European Enlightenment. In the 17th century, the philosophical dualism of Rene Descartes had posited an increasingly fragmented and discursive view of the human person, and the development of the first 'secular' hospitals in post-revolutionary France significantly changed the doctor–patient relationship, with the systematic movement from 'patient' to 'case' (Foucault 1973; Shorter 1993). This subversion of the doctor–patient relationship led, by way of germ, and then cell, theory in the 19th century and the development of molecular and nuclear medicine in the 20th, to the model of healthcare that has been characterised as the 'medical' or 'bio-medical' model. This reductionist and atomistic way of regarding the person regards human 'being' as no more than a biological phenomenon invaded by disease from the outside, causing changes in the body beyond the individual's control and making the body no more than the 'battleground' on which the doctor's 'war' on disease is waged, rather than the way in which the 'self' is presented to the world. This dominant and powerful discourse of disease predominated in medical practice and education until at least the last quarter of the 20th century when, having come under significant sociological, philosophical and even medical critique (Cassell 1991; Foucault 1973; Illich 1990), more holistic models re-emerged from more historic, and even ancient, characterisations of health, illness and the human person. These included what has been characterised as the bio-psycho-social model, first postulated by Engel (1962) in the early 1960s.

Cassell (1991) has argued cogently that with its focus on physical (bodily) pain, medicine was neglecting suffering, which, he argues, is not experienced simply in bodies but by persons and emerges when illness not only threatens the physical mechanism of the body but threatens the integrity of the person him or herself, seen as a whole. Indeed, Tom Driver (1991) regards suffering as a social performance that expresses the deep human search for meaning. Out of this re-integration of the self and the body, which Graham (1992) sees as 'the primary basis...for generating our sense of selfhood' (p.73) in which medical care is set within the context of concern for the whole person, including their wider life context, has come a rediscovery of the place of dialogue in which the narrative of the body is listened and responded to, so that the patient's voice is once again heard. Such listening, because it fundamentally attributes value or worth to the self and therefore recognises the obligation placed upon the listener, is itself a profoundly ethical act. Indeed, the *Encyclopedia of Ethics* (Montgomery 1979) suggests that one of the defining characteristics of the human species is its narrative nature and, as Arthur Frank (1995), a pioneer of modern narrative method, notes, 'in wounded story telling the physical act becomes the ethical act' (p.xii). Thus, spiritual care, narratively expressed, requires practitioners to have a person-centred rather than task-centred orientation and to remember that their language and their actions (both of which are communicative) will seldom, if ever, be, or be construed to be, value-free.

Robinson (2008) suggests that virtues are communicated through attentive listening to the stories of others and are modelled through the development of relationship. Thus the self, including the moral self, of both care-giver and care-receiver is profoundly engaged in the construction and delivery of spiritual care; practitioners, in whatever discipline, will need to be virtue led as well as technically proficient if they are to be genuinely other-orientated. Nonetheless, as Jack Coulehan (2005), reflecting on the culture of contemporary profit-driven medicine, has argued, its 'depleted moral imagination' has left the profession 'beset on all sides by the disappointment, dissatisfaction and misunderstanding of the people it is supposed to serve' (p.892). Thus he argues for the need for a rediscovery of the virtues in medicine and medical education since it is precisely the affirmation of the person, as (to use Martin Buber's characterisation; Buber 1944) a 'thou' rather than an 'it', which enables the dialogical engagement that confers on each individual the indispensable dignity of personhood that so many under conditions of illness feel to have been ignored, eroded or misplaced. Frank (1995) likewise notes how the temporarily broken down body (i.e. the body under the conditions of sickness) so often 'becomes an "it" to be cured', a diminished, even a lost, sense of self that needs to be reconstructed in the light of present circumstance. Such a self will never be the same as the one that has been 'lost' as such 'selfs' are progressive, constantly changing in the flux of experience. As McFadyen (1990) contends, the self must always transcend experience since 'there is always an "I" beyond the "I" of present experience' (p.100).

Meakin and Kirklin (2000), although in many ways critical of recent trends in medical education to engage with the humanities, comment that,

> these are exciting times for medical humanities in the UK, with artists and scientists working hand in hand to help deliver a more humanistic approach to health care… Specialists in literature, fine art, drama and medical history are bringing their expertise and enthusiasm to bear on the training of future health professionals. As a result productive and promising collaborations are taking place across traditional disciplinary boundaries. (Meakin and Kirklin 2000, p.49)

Whilst a lack of narrative acumen can be seen to have been systematically cultivated in medicine (Bleakley 2005), Rita Charon (2006), a physician with a doctorate in English and one of the pioneers of the use of narrative method in the practice and, particularly, the teaching of medicine, which she describes as 'medicine practiced with competence to recognise, absorb, interpret and be moved by stories of illness' (p.vii) says that, 'patients lament that their doctors don't listen to them or that they seem indifferent to their suffering. Fidelity and constancy seem to have become casualties of the cost-conscious bureaucratic marketplace' (p.3). She notes that 'sick people need physicians who can understand their diseases, treat their medical problems, and accompany them through their illness' but that 'a scientifically competent medicine alone cannot help a patient grapple with a loss of health or find meaning in suffering…physicians need the ability to listen to the narratives of the patient, grasp and honour their meanings, and be moved to act on the patient's behalf' (2001, p.1897).

Such practice makes medicine and wider healthcare an essentially relational project, rescuing medicine from the hegemony of technological dominance and restoring its place as a humane art. As Charon (2006) says, 'A medicine practiced without a genuine and obligating awareness of what patients go through may fulfil its technical goal, but it is an empty medicine, or, at best, half a medicine' (p.6). The dogged persistence of the epistemic distance increasingly created by post-enlightenment atomistic models, which reduce knowledge of the body to its parts rather than seeing it as an integrated whole, can be seen in recent developments in what has been characterised as 'stratified' or (ironically) 'personalised' medicine. The rise of bioinformatics, which, by combining anonymised medical information using mathematical algorithms and the consequent clustering of groups of patients to provide targeted medical care, has further alienated the patient as 'person' by creating another layer of distance in the doctor–patient relationship. Ironically, then, at the same time as medical technology has developed, and with it increased expectations of attaining a 'cure', the recipients of medical care have, in inverse proportion, become increasingly dissatisfied with the personal dimension of their care in which they feel neither 'heard' nor 'seen'. Emily Martin (1992) has suggested that this alienation is particularly acute for women, while Nell Noddings (1989) argues for the primacy of a relation ethic over individualistic ethics particularly to mitigate such alienation. She argues that such a relational ethic is predicated on shared human experience, particularly that of pain and suffering and arises out of a commitment to others in caring and being cared for.

The thrust of this section is to argue that in constructing spiritual care, the starting point is an understanding of health as a performed activity in which the needs of the sick person are best met by a dialogical, holistic, person-centred, multi-disciplinary approach, that engages both virtues and skills in reflective practice. In this, the critical questions of identity, relationality and care are addressed not merely as theoretical constructs but as part and parcel of lived human experience. As the phenomenologist Maurice Merleau-Ponty (1962) observed, 'Life is not what I think but what I live through' (p.xviii). This takes both effort and skill and the cultivation of an attitude that is essentially *agapeistic*, something that Alastair Campbell (1984) sees, in itself, as a way of 'knowing'. The philosopher Simone Weil (1951) wrote that, '(t)he capacity to give one's attention to a sufferer is a rare and difficult thing'(p.59). Whilst 'warmth of heart, impulsiveness and pity are not enough' she argues that such neighbour-love (*agape*) means being able to say to him or her, 'What are you going through?' (p.59). This 'extreme attention' to others is the essence of other-orientation and, Weil (1952) argues, taken to its highest degree, is the same thing as prayer. It presupposes faith and love. Similarly, Arthur Frank (1995) in his seminal work on narrative medicine asserts that 'one of our most difficult duties as human beings is to listen to the voices of those who suffer' and he concludes, as we have noted, that whilst 'listening is hard…it is also a fundamental moral act' (p.25). The Canadian ethicist, William May (1987) sees such care relationships as, by nature, 'covenantal' rather than 'contractual' since they are both gratuitous and involve a 'growing edge', which allows for the building of relationships. Elsewhere May (1996) argues that such a covenantal ethic 'defines the moral life responsively' (p.52). Such love confers value and is fundamental not only in Judeo-Christian ethics where it is intimately related to spiritual care, but even in secular moral codes where it may be implicit rather than explicit. Love, in this context, involves the virtue of fidelity that stays with the other in their vulnerability and is prepared to live non-judgementally with their fear, frustration, anxiety and (appropriately expressed) anger. When it becomes a component of change even existential anger can become an aspect of the healing process. Frances Young (1990) describes such anger as the 'dark side of love' (p.158) without which there is no hope of change. In his ethical analysis of agapeistic love, Gene Outka (1972, p.179), expresses it thus: 'Love does not snatch us from the pain of time, but takes the pain of the temporal upon itself. Hope makes us ready to bear the "cross of the present". It can hold to what is dead and hope for the unexpected' (p.179). It will sound strange, even counter-cultural, to some, especially to those schooled in 'professionalism' to speak of care in terms of love. Nonetheless, love and professionalism (in terms of acting professionally) are not mutually exclusive. Reinhold Niebuhr (1956) expresses it thus:

> *Love is reverence: It keeps its distance even as it draws near; it does not seek to absorb the other in the self or want to be absorbed by it; it rejoices in the otherness of the other; it desires the beloved to be what he is and does not seek to refashion him into a replica of the self or to make him a means of self-advancement. (Niebuhr 1956, p.35)*

Here we see a theological expression of a love that is genuinely 'other-regarding', that balances the intimacy and distance which are the hallmarks of professionalism in care, that is relational in form and content and seeks the well-being that is at the heart of all good, holistic, person-centred healthcare.

If Weil and Frank, Outka and Niebuhr are correct then constructing spiritual care, like other forms of care in the practice of medicine and healthcare in what Charon (2009) calls the 'glaring unclothing of illness' (p.118), are not simply intuitive. They require work – intellectual and emotional – to provide a robust, coherent, defensible and competent multi-disciplinary skill-set that can be applied consistently across healthcare systems.

The starting point for any such enterprise is the recognition that relationality is fundamentally constitutive of what it means to be human. This is true theologically, ethically and from the multi-disciplinary perspective of narrative medicine. Indeed, Charon (2006) speaks tellingly of the 'redemptive force' (p.80) of narrative itself to heal. Without relationality there can be no shared narrative, and the narrative in itself constitutes relationship – the shared story bridging the gap between teller and hearer, both of whom are needed to be authentically present in any such dynamic. Such stories are not only articulated verbally, but performed in and through the body since it is not only 'in' the body, as both self and not-self, that illness is localised, but 'through' the body that the self, not least the social self, is spoken and identity is formed or, to use McFadyen's (1990) characterisation, 'personhood', with all its multi-dimensionality, is 'sedimented'. For McFadyen, such existing-in-relationship is primarily dialogical. Embodiment is therefore a crucial dimension of personal being and relationality is the prerequisite for personhood (Kelly 1992;

McFayden 1990). Similarly, Larry Kent Graham (1992) argues that, 'the ministry of care requires a theory of personhood if it is to effectively increase the welfare of individuals and their communities' (p.70). Graham regards the self as 'a synthesis of values' (p.84) that is created and sustained by the connections of self with the world the self inhabits. Those who are well often have little need to talk about their bodies but for the sick person whose received sense of self and the horizons of whose world are often radically called into question by their condition, and for whom the world and their place within it is subject to re-interpretation, it is essential. Such interpersonal story-telling is fundamental in establishing identity, both personal and social, and in facilitating healing by bringing order out of the chaos of illness. As Christoph Schwobel (2006) observes, '(a) relational approach to the question of what it means to be human cannot ignore the question of our capacities and incapacities, nor indeed the question of our needs' (p.49). Thus, learning to listen to the narrative of the body and learning genuinely to 'hear' what the bodies of sick people are saying in the total ecology of treatment and thus allowing its externalisation, is the ineluctable starting point of constructing spiritual care. This is the case as much as it is in the practice of narrative medicine and the one has the capacity to inform and refine the other in the search for healing and wholeness. Dialogical relationality not only forms the basis of care in practice but is pivotal in our understanding of the way in which human identity, or personhood, is constructed and understood.

The recognition of the place of spirituality and of spiritual care in the practice of medicine is now well established. Before the turn of the 21st century the Director General of the World Health Organization (WHO 1998) had already recognised the subtle and broadening shifts in the understanding of medicine that were taking place. He wrote:

> *Until recently the health professions have largely followed a medical model, which seeks to treat patients by focussing on medicines and surgery, and gives less importance to beliefs and to faith. This reductionist or mechanistic view of patients as being only a material body is no longer satisfactory. Patients and physicians have begun to realise the value of elements such as faith, hope and compassion in the healing process. The value of such 'spiritual' elements in health and quality of life has led to research in this field in an attempt to move towards a more holistic view of health that includes a non-material dimension, emphasising the seamless connections between mind and body. (WHO 1998, cited in NHS Scotland 2009, p.7)*

The complex relationship between religious and spiritual care, often inaccurately used interchangeably, or worse still synonymously, is explored by Ferguson-Stuart in Chapter 2 of this book. Defining what is meant by words like 'spiritual' and 'spirituality' is notably difficult. What most definitions have in common, however, is the concept of relationality that is at the heart of this section on constructing spiritual care. Peter Speck (1988) – whose modelling of spiritual care is explored more fully in this section by Stephen Flatt (Chapter 3) – highlights the way in which relationship is essential in the sick person's search for meaning and becomes definitive for a developing spirituality. Thus spirituality, and spiritual care, which is its concomitant, involves people in assumptions both about how things are and how they ought to be, questions frequently raised in the context of illness or hospitalisation as the sick person seeks to bring meaning and coherence to their experience and to enhance their self-worth. Kitwood and Benson (1995) describe care, as defined above, as being 'concerned primarily with the maintenance and enhancement of personhood' (p.9).

It is because of this that the construction of narratives which give meaning to an individual's life-story is of such importance in the context of illness. They offer an orientation to the experience and allow the sick person to redraw their life-map bringing order back into the disorientating and disordering 'chaos' of the life-changing experience of illness. As such, it may be helpful to speak of spiritual care as enabling integration to re-emerge from the disintegration of the self (person) that the experience of illness so often precipitates. Spiritual care, therefore, has both an existential dimension in that it has the capacity to guide conduct in the present, and a transcendent dimension in that it relates the individual to that which is outside (or 'above' or 'beyond') the self. Theologically, this may be expressed in terms of there being both a horizontal and a vertical dimension to human personhood. Importantly, as it involves the whole person, including feelings, judgements, creativity and thinking, spirituality and spiritual care is both cognitive and affective and is subject to change and adaptation, not least as life experience and circumstances change through the experience of illness. This was something that Viktor Frankl (1962) noted over half a century ago in his book *Man's Search for Meaning*. He writes, 'The meaning of life differs from man to man, from day to day, from hour to hour. What matters, therefore, is not the meaning of life in general but rather the specific meaning of a person's life at a given moment' (p.130).

It is important to note that chaplains themselves need to learn how to 'construct' spiritual care as much as teaching others how to construct it. Elizabeth Kübler-Ross (1997), one of the pioneers of the hospice movement, has been critical of the failure of some chaplains in the past to move beyond 'religious' care to embrace a more inclusive 'spiritual' care. She writes,

> Over the years most of the people who have asked to speak to hospital chaplains had (sic.) been disappointed. 'All they want to do is read from their little black book', I heard repeatedly. In effect real questions had been sidestepped in place of some convenient quotation from the bible and a quick exit by the chaplain who was unsure of what to do. (Kübler-Ross 1997, p.149)

In Chapter 4 Anne McCormick demonstrates how a narrative and dialogical use of, and engagement with, scripture can be used much more profitably in the construction and delivery of spiritual care.

As with the word 'spiritual', the word 'care' also requires more critical definition. If 'care', as 'being with' another and therefore open to their reality is important, then 'caring', including spiritual caring, involves both virtues and skills. Since, I have argued, love (*agape*) is the underpinning quality of the spiritual care relationship, spiritual care is at heart both social and relational. This is why I argue in this chapter that it is important to resist the medicalisation of spiritual care. This reduces 'spiritual distress' to a diagnosable and assessable phenomenon, which takes it outside the interpersonal dynamic since spiritual care and spiritual well-being are not simply a matter of psychological adjustment but of an intrinsically existential reorientation in which the spiritual care-giver is best described as 'accompanist'. The restructuring of the care relationship in terms of 'being' rather than 'doing' may do much to mitigate the 'fix-it', problem solving mentality that has permeated so much of contemporary healthcare and has led to the target-driven culture that has so frustrated both care-receivers and care-givers, a fact explored by Flatt in his section on staff morale in Chapter 3.

What is it that provides the distinctive for spiritual care in the overall economy of patient-centred, whole-person care? First of all, there is context since chaplains as the primary though not sole deliverers of spiritual care often have by virtue of their role the time to listen to and engage with the stories of others in a way that busy physicians, held as they are in the thrall of target-driven bureaucracies, have not. Second, the long history of engagement with narrative by those who inhabit the spiritual traditions of faith communities gives them an informed familiarity with the use of narrative with which practitioners within other disciplines, especially those characterised as more 'scientific' (which does not necessarily imply being more 'objective', 'critical' or 'evidence-based') have only more recently begun to engage. Third, an increased engagement with academic and cross-disciplinary research into spiritual care, to provide a robust theoretical underpinning to inform practice serves to inform the practice and delivery of a holistic, person-centred healthcare that is now irreducibly interdisciplinary. As Gaylord Noyce (1989) notes, 'the most useful theological reflection takes place in dialogue with practice' (p.21).

At the heart of good healthcare is the developed capacity for skilled and attentive interpersonal communication, which, when set alongside spiritual care, as Gordon, Kelly and Mitchell (2011) note, together go 'beyond information giving and are firmly rooted in the "personal" part of interpersonal' (p.22). Thus medicine that is genuinely person-centred and that takes spiritual and religious care seriously in the economy of care is predicated on the recognition of, and respect for, the unique 'otherness' of each person. In the context of such an authentic and empathetic care-receiver/care-giver dynamic both parties are engaged, intellectually and emotionally, opened to the possibility of change, the gap between individuals is narrowed and the humanity of each emerges. It is here that the role of narrative comes into its own. As Rita Charon (2001) notes, 'by bridging the divide that separates the physician from the patient, the self, colleagues, and society, narrative medicine can help physicians offer accurate, engaged, and effective care of the sick' (p.1901). Sayantani DasGupta (2003, 2008) observes how, whilst the practice of medicine and healthcare is concerned with the bodies of others, its practitioners, whether doctors or chaplains, seldom have (or perhaps make) the time to explore their own bodily experiences. In and of itself, this exacerbates the imbalance in the relationship of care.

Anne McCormick opens Chapter 4 in this volume with the words, 'Chaplains are by default interpreters...' Interpretation is an act that requires both attentive listening to words, whether spoken or written, and reflection, and it is in the multi-layered interplay between these (what theologians, especially in their description of the dynamic relationships expressed within the doctrine of the Trinity, characterise as *perichoresis*), and between 'self' and 'other' that interpretation takes place. In this process, the role of imagination, an essential element in creative story-making, is key. It would be a fundamental mistake, however, to confuse such creative story-making with fantasy, the associative with the dissociative – on the contrary, such profound narrative story-making engages lived reality at its deepest level and requires the rigorous and critical application of both rationality and intuition. As Miriam Solomon (2008) perceptively observes, '(n)arrative medicine is not unreflective story-telling or feel-good group therapy for health-care providers' (p.412). Within the context of healthcare structures, Bob Whorton (2011) offers the insightful observation that, properly understood, '(t)he NHS work-culture today desperately needs the resources of imagination. A cold bureaucratic, target driven approach leaves us at best uninspired and at worst resistant and angry' (p.22). McCormick, writing from a mental health perspective, explores the use of the Bible as an interpretive tool, recognising that for chaplains, their identification with their own faith narrative itself informs their responses to service-users, in what Ferguson-Stuart in Chapter 2 characterises as 'the practice and narrative of faith'. In this dynamic both care-receivers and care-givers, through both what they say and do – for narrative is, as we have seen, 'performed' as well as spoken, become what Rita Charon (2005) describes as 'obligatory story-tellers and story-listeners' (p.261). Charon (2009) herself recognises the role played by theology and she acknowledges that, '(m)y flight of ideas into Christian theology helped me to visualise and recognise that the patient, in my office, exists plurally' (p.124).

In the report, 'Spiritual care matters' (NHS Scotland 2009) we find the following assertion:

> Spiritual care in the NHS must be both inclusive and accepting of human difference. As we learn to listen better to the particular needs of different people, so we equip ourselves for work that is more fulfilling and effective. The provision of spiritual care by NHS staff is not yet another demand on their hard pressed time. It is the essence of their work and enables and promotes healing in the fullest sense to all parties, both giver and receiver of such care. (NHS Scotland 2009, p.1)

Best practice in care, and not least in the construction of spiritual care, is therefore person-centred rather than problem-centred, holistic rather than atomistic in its understanding of human being. It is interdisciplinary and cooperative rather than parochial and competitive in its approach and, above all, it is genuinely *agapeistic*. Furthermore, since it is grounded in love, such faithful presence before the other creates and sustains genuine community. It is now nearly half a century since the American ethicist Paul Ramsey (1970) wrote his seminal book, *The Patient as Person*. In it, Ramsey uses the concept of 'person' as a Kantian counterbalance to modern medicine's tendency to maximise benefits, whether knowledge or life. Since then, such 'benefits' have become increasingly technological and financial and the losers have all too often been the very ones that healthcare services purport to serve. The words of Seneca with which this chapter opened serve as a timely reminder that the focus of healthcare is not, or at least ought not to be, either 'targets' or 'outcomes' in and of themselves, but rather the patient as person, complex, vulnerable, fragmented but ultimately capable of the wholeness, individual and social, that healing brings.

Note

1.   *Non tamquam amicus videt sed tamquam **imperator*** (my emphasis) – 'one who commands', that is, as a client.

CHAPTER 2

Discourses of Spiritual Healthcare

Hamish Ferguson-Stuart

Introduction

It would be difficult to work in the modern NHS without hearing
spirituality mentioned, or meeting a widespread acceptance of the
discourse of spirituality among healthcare professionals. Paradoxically,
chaplains, the group specifically charged with meeting the need for
religious and spiritual care may feel some unease. The root of this
lies not in the welcome recognition that the spiritual is a vital part
of holistic care, but in the difference between the spirituality implicit
in healthcare usage and the spirituality accepted in the traditions
from which chaplains are drawn. To distinguish between these two
understandings in what follows, I retain lower case for the former, but
capitalise the latter.

This chapter focuses on that difference and its relevance to and
implications for chaplains. My aim is threefold: to show that a knowledge
of the discourse gives chaplains insight into the culture within which
they work; that the theological resources available to chaplains offer a
vantage point from which to critique spirituality; and, finally, to suggest
this discourse of spirituality also interrogates chaplains. What sort of
theology might be both truthful and audible in the healthcare setting?

Seeking to account for the strong and widespread acceptance of
spirituality in healthcare, I examine, first, its genesis and congruence
with themes that are an integral part of the distinctive subculture
of healthcare. This can give spirituality an air of overwhelming
inevitability; to moderate this impression, I then turn to more critical
voices. Although the institutional culture of healthcare appears
homogenous, it is full of contradictions and ambiguities; a purportedly

homogenous secular arena both publicly and privately interlaced with the sacred. This ambiguity is fully shared by spirituality, so I consider next those critiques that argue against its validity, necessity or adequacy; paradoxically these too are part of the discourse.

The final section is a reflection on spirituality, from the viewpoint of a practising Anglican chaplain in acute healthcare but with the advantage of having inhabited the changing culture of the NHS since the early 1970s. As a nurse for over 30 years many of the pressures and incidents in the following pages resonate with my own experience, and elicit my sympathy.

The discourse of spirituality
The development of the discourse

Forty years ago, the medical paradigm dominated healthcare. It supplied professional and epistemological standards to which other healthcare professions aspired, and in day-to-day healthcare provided ways of relating to patients and their illnesses. As experienced by a patient, this medical model was instrumental, reductionist, generalising and abstracting. The vivid experience of illness was reinterpreted and rephrased in a vocabulary that was general, linking all similar experiences; reduced to abstract physical or anatomical concepts; the effect was depersonalising, suppressing individuality. Care language was not expressed in the language of 'they *have*, but the ontological statement they *are*' (Swift 2001, p.103, emphasis original). It was a process that, once experienced, was seldom forgotten. To some degree it was inherent in the instrumental model of healthcare, affecting the attitudes of healthcare professionals to their patients. '(S)taff treated him as an object they had to treat rather than a human being who should be included in his care and given the dignity that he deserves' (The Patients' Association 2011, p.13).

A further effect of such a system was to render invisible the experiences and concepts that could not be reframed in the medical vocabulary: there were no professional words enabling a caring response to the uncertainty, distress and grief that often accompany illness, or to the philosophical and theological issues of justice and theodicy raised by illness.

When the NHS was founded, these questions and fears would have been considered the chaplain's province. Two factors changed this. One was the decreasing familiarity of religion, its practices and narratives, to large sections of society. It became harder to relate the practice and narratives of faith to personal experience of illness. Indeed many had contact with religion only in the context of death and funerals – an association making ministers, priests – or chaplains – seem inappropriate providers of support to the living.

Second, and more pragmatically, although chaplains were part of the NHS since its inception, most chaplaincy until the late 1980s was provided by visiting parochial clergy and ministers, a situation described by Child (1965). Aside from considerations of easy availability, chaplains rarely became familiar and accepted participants (however marginally) in the quotidian life of healthcare. The task of responding to spiritual need or distress was therefore increasingly thrown on staff; principally on nurses.

And those needs persisted. McSherry records an instance (2007, pp.171–172) in which a devout Roman Catholic patient did not receive the sacraments before his death, a matter of great importance to him and his family. The resultant haunting sense of failing a patient kindled McSherry's interest in spiritual care; he has become a major contributor to the area since.

More widely, the last 30 years have seen a major shift in the content of spirituality. Within the UK this could be summarised as a separating of spirituality from its roots in a specific tradition and praxis, a minimising of the differences between religions and emphasis on shared insights that could be separated from their origins and recombined into an eclectic, self-constructed spirituality, focusing on personal aspirations, self-fulfilment and integration, of inner peace within an immanent matrix.

These factors, the felt need for a framework within which healthcare professionals could offer spiritual support and the plausibility of such a framework came together in the discourse of spiritual care. Given their greater contact with patients, this was perhaps most apparent to nurses; certainly they have been at the forefront in its development over the last 30 years, but many other healthcare professionals have been drawn into it. A prodigious number of papers, articles and books have appeared; but implicit in them is a particular form of spirituality, to whose salient features I now turn.

The shape of a spirituality

A spirituality that attempts to be applicable to all is necessarily a wide-ranging, protean concept, difficult to define. Nonetheless, many were offered. They offered ready critical targets, as Swinton (2006) points out, for their lack of an empirical basis, the wideness of the boundaries they drew, their attempts to smuggle religious categories of thought into a secular arena, and their meaninglessness and fatuity. More tellingly, they seemed divorced from practice. How can one move from a vague definition to the spiritual care of a distressed patient? With the turn of the century, the emphasis moved from definition to actual giving of spiritual care. Participants in the discourse, instead of trying to define boundaries turned instead to analysing its typical features. Thus,

> *Members of the exploring spirituality groups that I worked with discussed a number of definitions of spirituality...but remained reluctant to define spirituality too closely themselves. We preferred to identify key themes and concepts that could be used to describe and explore spirituality. (White 2006, p.84)*

White goes on to provide a typical and convenient list:

Spirituality is...

- An innate potential in every person
- Unique to each individual
- The essence of being human
- Integrated not separated from body and mind
- Transcendent but not separated from body and mind
- To be nurtured
- Linked to meaning, hope and connection with others
- Not the same as religion, although it might be linked.

(White 2006, p.86)

It is easier, and more practical, to consider the mechanics of spiritual care, what interventions on the part of healthcare practitioners are needed, from such a list. But even so providing spiritual care was not trouble free. In 2008 Caroline Petrie, a nurse, was suspended from duty because she had offered to pray for a patient. The incident led to widespread debate in the healthcare professions and criticism of the guidance on spiritual care, or lack of it, available to nurses and other healthcare professionals.

In 2010 the Royal College of Nursing (RCN) launched a survey of its members' views on 'spirituality and spiritual care in nursing practice'. The following year, the RCN issued a guide to 'spirituality and nursing care' with a list of the features of spiritual care that parallels White's.

Spirituality is about:

- hope and strength

- trust

- meaning and purpose

- forgiveness

- belief and faith in self, others, and for some this includes a belief in a deity/higher power

- peoples' values

- love and relationships

- morality

- creativity and self expression.

(Royal College of Nursing 2011, p.4)

As well as this list of what it considers to be the salient points of spirituality, the pamphlet offers helpful advice on discerning the need for spiritual care and its practice. There is also a section on what spiritual care is not, emphasising that it is not 'about imposing your own beliefs and values on another' or 'using your position to convert' (Royal College of Nursing 2011, p.5).

Comparing these two lists, several themes emerge. There is the stress on the autonomous individual (though slightly mitigated by the acknowledgement of the importance of love and relationships in the RCN's formulation) and meaning as something essential to a purposeful human life. There is the separation of spirituality and religion; they may or may not be linked.

All this relates closely to the subculture of healthcare and the wider culture of the society of which it is a part; the importance of personal autonomy and informed choice, the analytical approach to spirituality, breaking it into smaller units in the search to discover what it is and an emphasis on the conceptual and the intellectual. Religion is a matter of private choice, different to spirituality. There is a hint of the distrust of religion, common after the events of 9/11 in 2001 and reinforced by subsequent terrorist attacks. This distrust identified religion with political extremism and terrorism; religion becomes threatening and untrustworthy, a source of violence, a view which seemed to reach its apogee in the handbook *Religion or Belief: A Practical Handbook for the NHS* (Department of Health 2009). There the subtext seemed almost to read 'spirituality good, religion bad'.

All these features parallel closely the deepest assumptions of the healthcare subculture, the place of the 'implicit assumptions that actually guide behaviour, that tell group members how to perceive, think about, and feel about things' (Schein 1985, p.18). It affects profoundly what can be said, how the world and human potential are viewed and what is considered plausible and valid.

Also implicit here is the assumption that this is a homogenous subculture. Certainly this assumption is encouraged by such central government documents as the NHS Constitution (Department of Health 2012). But this is far from the case, as O'Neill (2013, p.17) notes. Local cultures reflecting the history of particular hospitals are cross-cut by professional and vocational subcultures. These cultural cross-currents and oppositions also affect how the spiritual care is put into practice.

One point where this more complex picture comes to the surface is the apparent clear separation between secular healthcare and religious belief. This seems ironic given the historical links between the sacred and care of the sick and on closer examination proves to be not entirely accurate. The next section, then, considers this in more detail.

The cultural matrix
Religious and secular in healthcare
Such a separation would have seemed strange to some of the most influential figures in healthcare's history. Florence Nightingale, who, however her career is interpreted, remains a major figure in the history and identity of modern nursing, wrote that 'God spoke to me and called me to his service' (Baly 1991, p.18). A similar sense of calling, of vocation, was a factor – often a major one – leading many to enter healthcare professions. Though less so than in the past, I would suggest, drawing on personal experience and conversation, religious factors continue to be an important source of inspiration among

health professionals. The vision of meeting Christ in the care of the sick (Matthew 25:36) remains powerful in the professional lives of many in the healthcare world. Simultaneously, the working out of this vision often has difficulties. Whipp (1999) draws attention to conflicts that can arise when a fundamentally religious vocation is worked out in the secular arena, conflicts even more dramatically illustrated by the case of Caroline Petrie, as noted earlier.

Despite the importance of religious ideals in healthcare, and the support of the churches for it, the NHS originated in a vision of a (secular) 'New Jerusalem' (discussed in Barnett 2001, pp.125–139). Yet this secular institution continues to provide chapels and quiet spaces for prayer and reflection, public and private. From its inception it has employed chaplains and called them to publicly mark events in the institution's life – memorials, dedications, occasions of remembrance. It is an institution of paradoxes that runs throughout its life.

The setting: Ambiguities and paradoxes

Some of the deepest roots of NHS culture lie in the enlightenment project. This carries with it a group of unexamined, rarely articulated assumptions: the centrality of the autonomous individual and the primacy of instrumental rationality by which an accurately planned future can be attained, a primacy currently reinforced by the ascendency of managerial modes of thought and practice. Coupled with these is a distrust of and aversion to tradition – a conviction that human life takes place in an immanent world, from which the transcendent has been banished. Here, religion becomes a private matter, excluded, or at best marginal to the public space of discourse.

This is articulated through a distinctive use of language, which aspires to simplicity, clarity and precision. The extensive technical vocabulary of medicine, intended for precision, is a good example of this. There is little place here for analogy and metaphor, the staples of poetic thought – and of spiritual discourse in religious traditions. This specialised language clothes a way of thinking and understanding that is radically analytic, breaking things and situations down into smaller units in the search for the understanding that will give control. Definitions are important, establishing the precise meanings of phenomena; enabling them to be incorporated and manipulated in a rational discourse.

Many of these features can be discerned in the discourse of spirituality; the same centrality of the individual exists in a world devoid, for all practical purposes, of the transcendent – except as a private option. There is the same stress on practicality, on meaning attained by rational thinking and autonomous choice. But, as elsewhere, we are not talking about an entirely homogenous way of regarding the world. Non-instrumental language and metaphorical and analogical modes of discourse persist in surprising places.

This situation is epitomised in an assertion at the beginning of such a basic document as the NHS Constitution; the NHS 'works at the limits of science – bringing the highest levels of human knowledge and skill to save lives and improve health. It touches our lives at times of basic human need, when care and compassion are what matter most' (Department of Health 2012, p.2). The first sentence, with its references to 'science', 'knowledge' and 'skill', suggests a reliance on qualities attained by analysis, separation. Against this is balanced the insistence on relationship and compassion in the second sentence – an acknowledgement of the limitations of instrumentality and an appeal to qualities that sit more easily within the Christian than the enlightenment tradition.

This sums up neatly the complexities of NHS culture. The whole – and the spiritual care that is part of it – might be regarded as a conversation between different voices. Some of these voices are far more critical than others; it is to these that I turn.

Dissident voices

Stringent critiques of spirituality have been offered from both theological and secular stances. The arguments of the former will emerge in the next, and penultimate, section of this chapter; here I consider the secular critique. In one basic way it differs from other contributions to the discourse, because it argues strongly that there is no need for the discourse at all; that it is, indeed, illegitimate in the secular space of the NHS.

One prominent writer who takes this view (Paley 2008) begins by interrogating the available definitions of spirituality – the number of them and variety of them. In this he follows a common critical strategy, noted earlier, but follows this by questioning whether spirituality is really such an essential part of being human as its advocates assume.

In denying this he can, after all, draw on personal introspection and the opinion of others. This move enables him to argue that, consequently, it is not an essential aspect of healthcare. Does it meet any need that could not be met equally well by medicine, pharmacology or psychology – or even philosophy?

He goes on to suggest 'spirituality' is a ploy to smuggle the transcendent into an inappropriate forum, the secular space of healthcare. He responds by proposing to 'simply cancelling, perhaps one might say "bracketing" the inflated non-naturalistic claims [i.e. the transcendent] I have been discussing, in order to see what the spirituality terrain looks like from the naturalistic point of view' (p.9).

This tactic frees him from the need to counter the direct experience of healthcare professionals (including the author) that there is indeed a need for spiritual care. It also obviates the necessity of entering the far more complex debate about the relationship of the transcendent to the immanent or why the transcendent appears in a secular institution in a secular society at all. Moreover, prescinding from the transcendent frees him to raise questions about the motivation of the discourse – is the driving force behind this discourse a desire for the enhancement of nurses' professional status more than a felt patient need? Whilst this may be one possible explanation of the discourse, it seems too frail to bear the weight it is being asked to carry. It also overlooks the extent to which the discourse of spiritual care involves members of other healthcare professions.

However the argument enables the focus to be shifted to larger issues: political and economic themes addressing the 'spirituality' current in wider society. Paley follows Carrette and King (2005) in construing it as a power game designed to produce docile subjects and consumers; providing them with responses to an encouraged need, to which religion is no longer a plausible answer, generating a potentially lucrative market.

Undoubtedly some of Paley's criticisms are timely: many theologians would agree with his strictures on the fatuity of many constructions of spirituality, and his thoughts about the role of professional aggrandisement are a timely caution. However, his thesis as a whole seems insufficient to account for the widespread interest in spirituality in healthcare. His careful 'bracketing' of transcendence, particularly, leaves the reader feeling the discourse of spirituality has been explained away rather than explained.

A chaplain's reflections

The interest in spiritual care is very welcome to a chaplain, but for a chaplain, the spirituality implicit in this interest is difficult to accept uncritically. There is too much difference between spirituality and Spirituality for that. Three areas stand out; how professional habits carry over into spiritual care; second, the use of language in which that spirituality is articulated; and finally, the 'thinness' of that language.

PROFESSIONAL HABITS AND GIVING SPIRITUAL CARE

The discourse presupposes that spiritual support is an integral part of healthcare. But healthcare professionals attempting this bring with them the habits acquired during their professional lifetimes, so internalised that their presence is unsuspected, their effect automatic. Thus, the patient is seen, in effect, as an aggregation of various physiological systems rather than an integral whole. It is all too easy to regard the 'spiritual' as another such system. It may malfunction, leading to spiritual distress, a 'problem' to be solved by professional expertise.

But that expertise depends on there being a body of knowledge accepted as valid and applicable by patient and professional alike. In a non-religious, privatised spirituality, no such shared body of knowledge exists. Indeed, even within a private spirituality there may be contradictory currents. Famously, over 70 years ago, C.S. Lewis noted ironically 'Your man has been accustomed, ever since he was a boy, to have a dozen incompatible philosophies dancing about together inside his head' (Lewis 1942, p.11). If that was so then, it is even more so now, when 'even the most stable and homogenous societies have discovered that they already incorporate a degree of ontological pluralism that would have been difficult for Lewis (or even Screwtape) to foresee' (Prickett 2002, p.6).

Conceptualising spiritual distress as a 'problem' is itself problematic. It implies a definite and complete answer that returns the situation to what it was before. This may be impossible. In illness spiritual distress originates in the collision of the person with the limits of human finitude. In a non-theistic spirituality orientated towards self-fulfilment and integration, a terrifying experience even in a theistic tradition triggering an existential terror, a reaction well documented in the narratives of scripture (cf. Genesis 28:16–19). Such an encounter may not, of course, be terrifying, but an occasion of wonder and amazement pointing towards the infinite. 'Problem', however fixed in healthcare usage seems far too narrow a category to accommodate all this.

Even if spiritual care could be reduced to the application of specialised knowledge and technique it would differ from the chaplain's experience of spiritual care as a shared journey, a process affecting both giver and recipient, with all the risks to professional self-understanding and comfort that may bring.

Finally, professional interventions are instrumental by their very nature: they aim at a goal and have an intended outcome. They overlook the paradox of inattention. The simplest example of this is the common experience of being unable to bring a word to mind, no matter how hard one tries. Indeed, the harder one tries, the less likely it is that the word will come to mind. It is only when the attention has shifted to something else, and the difficulty is no longer in the conscious mind, that the missing word saunters into view, as though it had never been absent. Shaw (1988) draws attention to the way in which religious – and other – traditions use this paradox, reaching 'a goal by giving up the attempt to reach it' (p.1). But this idea is very difficult to accept within an instrumental milieu, where focus on outcomes and goals, inseparable from current healthcare practice, potentially inhibits rather than facilitates relief of spiritual distress.

THE USE OF LANGUAGE

To a chaplain, the spirituality assumed in the literature seems excessively verbal and conceptual. Moreover, the language itself is 'thin'; with no depth of meaning or allusion. One reason is the lack of a shared, reflectively developed tradition and narrative: but it is not helped by the way in which language is used in the discourses of healthcare. As hinted at earlier, language here is a careful descriptive matter, where it is important that a word refers to one thing, and one thing only. Whilst this may be necessary in an analytical mode of forming meaning, language in religious traditions is rather different. What appear to be plain narratives are marked by what might be called a poetic use of language. Words are valued precisely because they are not exact, but always come with a number of associations. Especially where words are used analogically this enables connections to be made, meaning found and a picture built up that points beyond the present, perhaps distressing, situation.

Language used in this way also draws on the strength of metaphor, where image meets lived experience as 'words are used so as to activate a broad net of connotations, which, though present to us, remains implicitly so' (McGilchrist 2009, p.115). Admittedly, healthcare has inherited the Enlightenment's suspicion of metaphor – though using it readily enough for persuasive ends. But effective spiritual care at times hinges on the discovery and development in conversation of a resonant metaphor for the patient's situation. To persons habituated to this poetic usage, the familiar texts of a religious tradition possess an apparently inexhaustible depth and applicability to present need. It leaves the conceptual, far more literal discourse of spirituality, thin and arid by contrast.

'THINNESS'; SHARED AND FRAGMENTED NARRATIVES

Interestingly, a similar 'thinness' can be observed in contemporary characterisations of religion: 'a religion is a belief system with no basis in reality whatever. Religious belief is without reason and without dignity, and its record is near-universally dreadful' (Martin Amis, quoted in Beattie 2007, p.3). This is an extreme view, of surprising historical naiveté; more common is the assumption that religion is a collection of beliefs that are tacked onto a secular word view. The more accurate view, that a religious tradition offers ways of looking at and understanding the world, is below the horizon. Religion is presumed to exist within the person, rather than the person being formed within the religious tradition.

A central feature of spirituality is the emphasis it places on meaning as necessary to spiritual health and resilience. The view parallels the high regard given to knowledge in secular culture:

> *Indeed, a great part of the excitement of life in the post-Enlightenment period has come with the thought that reality could be reconceived, that knowledge would emancipate humankind, if only it could be made accessible to them. (Robinson 2010 p.3)*

This is a very high view of knowledge: operating at the deepest level of healthcare culture, it might go some way towards explaining the centrality of meaning in spirituality.

But what meaning is, or how it may be found, is an enigma. The thrust of the discourse suggests it is a matter of free choice. But it then follows, given the current distrust of tradition, that it will be developed from what is currently available, limited by criteria of fashion, social acceptability and personal preference. In this it differs from tradition, which is a given. Further, a tradition has a history; the insights and blind spots of one generation are balanced by the different insights and blind spots of others. Traditions play host to a multitude of voices, with different interests, abilities and approaches. The result is a density of reference and possibilities able to provide support at times of crisis in a way in which chosen meaning cannot. Choice, after all, is interior to the person, held onto by an act of will. Choices made can be unmade and, the will sapped by illness, may simply slip away. Chosen meaning does not have tradition's stability, exterior to the person. Moreover, major traditions are polyphonic: there are few situations they have not encountered and developed responses to.

Significance would be a more natural word for a chaplain in this context, rather than meaning. The sign, after all, points to something outside itself. In a Christian setting, this would include, ultimately a relationship with God. To the secular view this perhaps introduces a level of uncertainty, a loss of control ascribed to the individual that is hard to accept. Uncertainty does not fit well in healthcare culture, especially when the medical and managerial models dominate.

A religious Spirituality may better accommodate failure and mortality: here the self exists, as it were, in a more expansive setting. A culture formed by Enlightenment optimism and suffused by instrumentality has difficulty in accepting that tragedy and futility are inherent possibilities of the human condition, which cannot always be avoided, prevented or cured. Whilst any spiritual care in these circumstances will not be easy, a purely secular spirituality perhaps faces more difficulties, has less to offer, its 'thin' language hardly reflecting the gravity of situations it faces.

I have written as if secular and religious views of spirituality were easily distinguished, dialectical alternatives. As the brief survey of the complexity of healthcare culture offered in a previous section might suggest, this is a gross simplification; the reality is often far more fragmented, an inarticulate reaching for meaning and significance in the face of trauma. The picture here is of flowers left at the scene of a road accident.

Conclusion

Healthcare can be a place of marginalisation for any chaplain. Knowledge of the culture is essential; it enables the chaplain to relate to staff, to their stresses and strains. This is invaluable in pastoral contacts with staff, but also enables reflection and critique from the inside. That knowledge enables a realisation of how diverse the organisational culture is; how the chaplain is one voice among many. But a chaplain also represents a tradition, enabling reflections that are not only culturally relevant, but also have the critical distance and new insights stemming from a different tradition of understanding human purpose and possibility. It seems important, if this is to be maintained, that the roots of chaplaincy within the traditions of faith are carefully maintained and nurtured.

This is to say that what the chaplain is, is as important to him or her as knowledge and action. This might indicate an interesting convergence between spirituality and Spirituality: witness an intriguing, if undeveloped note in the RCN's guidance that spiritual care 'is about our attitudes, behaviours and our personal qualities i.e. how we are with people' (Royal College of Nursing 2011).

The discourse of spirituality also interrogates chaplains. What sort of theology might be both truthful and audible in the healthcare setting? This is too big a question to be answered here, but some salient features of it might be discerned. It would be relational, both in the immanent and transcendent frame, it would be panentheistic, conscious of the presence of God in and beyond all things, taking a contemplative stance, and finally, it would give full weight to the apophatic. It would need to be a humble theology, in the full sense of most unfashionable of qualities; not in the false sense of self-denigration, but in the true sense of clear awareness of what is, and a willingness to work with it. Such a theology might indeed be of great value to healthcare chaplains enabling the resources of tradition to be deployed in an arena of need.

CHAPTER 3

Making Use of Models of Healthcare Chaplaincy

Stephen Flatt

Introduction

'Models are not reality but they are a way of representing aspects of reality in a simplified form that allow us to explore and safely try out features of the world we live in' (Cobb 2004, p.14). Healthcare chaplaincy models provide a systematic approach to the work of chaplaincy departments; setting out a structured description of what happens and why it happens in this way. A documented approach provides a baseline against which the service can be measured and enables audit and research. Chaplaincy departments need to demonstrate that they are working from a strong evidence base and can provide proof of efficacy if they are to be taken seriously. 'The "journey" through the healthcare service requires an evidence base to show both what happens and that what happens is valuable in terms of intended outcomes and enhanced well-being' (Mowat 2008, p.72).

Healthcare chaplaincy is difficult to quantify; it deals with the spiritual, the pastoral and the religious, which may appear nebulous and ethereal – even marginal or niche. Where do chaplains fit in the work of the multi-disciplinary healthcare team; is their contribution of any significance? Without an understanding of chaplaincy's contribution to holistic healthcare it is difficult for those who commission and those who provide healthcare services to realise chaplaincy's true value.

Chaplaincy models are theoretical constructs that can enable healthcare organisations, practitioners, patients and the public to understand the organisation and work of healthcare chaplaincy. Models can reveal the intrinsic significance of spiritual health and well-being, as a part of holistic patient-centred healthcare, and its effect on things such as positive healthcare experience, patient satisfaction and staff morale. These have a real value in financial terms for trust governing bodies: shorter length of stay; improved organisational reputation; and lower staff sickness, absence and turnover are all ways of reducing costs and increasing income.

A better understanding of chaplaincy helps practitioners to make more informed referral and use of chaplaincy services; this enables resources to be used most effectively. Robust models of healthcare chaplaincy describe to colleagues how to make the most out of the chaplaincy services offered. They should also enable them to better understand their own role in spiritual care, or at least to realise that they have one.

Chaplaincy models are a means of expressing a theological understanding of health and healing in a more generally accessible medium. Models can highlight the search for meaning and purpose; the need to understand human experience within a transcendent reality, and at the same time more intimate spiritual needs such as companionship, forgiveness and love. Autton commenting on the ministry of hospital chaplaincy writes,

> Here is a challenge to every priest, for no ministry can be more full of opportunity, and none more meaningful and satisfying. Such a calling demands sharing the unsharable; entering into the very heart of shattering pain with something more shattering still. (Autton 1966, p.4)

The current challenge in the multi-faith and, at the same time, increasingly secular context in which most chaplaincies operate is to develop models that theologically embrace different understandings of the purpose and place of God in health and healing and with which the adherents of different faiths and those of no faith at all can identify (whilst maintaining the distinctiveness and integrity of each).

The context of healthcare chaplaincy in the NHS

The NHS came into being on 5 July 1948 with the vision of being a 'cradle to grave service' free at the point of delivery for all. There was a real belief that the nation could be freed from the scourge of sickness with programmes of education, vaccination and the use of new drugs such as antibiotics and diuretics. However, it is clear to even the casual observer that the NHS has changed almost beyond recognition over the last seven decades, not least because it was founded on what proved to be a flawed premise that, as the nation's health improved, demand on the service would fall.

Treating patients as individuals, listening to individual needs and involving them in decisions about care are all extremely positive advances in healthcare philosophy. However, with the NHS serving an increasingly diverse society, the attempt to meet the many different cultural, religious and spiritual needs of patients, families and staff becomes an ever increasing challenge. Recognising the spiritual and religious demands of all means not only being aware of 'mainstream' faiths but also taking into account myriad competing demands from a whole plethora of New Religious Movements and personal spiritualities.

Within three years of the inception of the NHS it was necessary to start charging for prescriptions and dental care and the cost of healthcare has continued to increase; an ageing population and advances in technology and treatments have cost implications. Every year services and departments are asked to make cost improvements and efficiencies and each must be able to demonstrate that they are good value for money; for many chaplaincy departments this scrutiny is a new experience. 'Caring for the spirit' (South Yorkshire Workforce Development Confederation 2003, p.18) speaks of the need to increase chaplaincy research to evidence the 'efficacy of spiritual healthcare'.

Advances in healthcare technology and treatments have changed the face of hospital care; length of stay has been reduced, the hospital population is more acutely unwell. The creation of centres of excellence and greater specialisation of healthcare services mean that patients and their relatives frequently travel long distances from home to receive tertiary and quaternary care. Sickness and hospital admission can engender a sense of isolation, and the physical distance from home and family multiplies this effect.

The increasingly high acuity and dependency of patients can have a negative impact on staff satisfaction and levels of stress; in this environment staff support is an increasingly pertinent and valuable role for chaplains to undertake. 'Professional chaplains play an important role in helping staff…their supportive consultation can enhance morale and decrease staff burnout, thus reducing employee turnover and the use of sick time' (VandeCreek and Burton 2001, p.15).

Healthcare delivery is changing; there is greater emphasis on community services and preventing or minimising hospital admissions.

Hospitals are getting smaller as beds are cut and the focus of care is moving from inpatient to outpatient, from treatment to prevention. Chaplains have the opportunity to work with their faith communities to build strong professional relationships and develop care pathways and competencies that ensure seamless, high quality, religious and spiritual healthcare for all in both the hospital and community setting.

Models of healthcare chaplaincy

Robust models of healthcare chaplaincy are essential in demonstrating how the service is addressing these challenges and remains a vital part of healthcare provision. A review of some of the common themes in chaplaincy models developed by Autton, Woodward, Speck, Wilson and Cobb over the last half century will be useful in informing the design of future healthcare chaplaincy models. As well as examining the themes in these models, consideration of generic chaplaincy as a potential model will prove helpful.

The distinctive nature of chaplaincy and the pastoral relationship

Norman Autton, in his 1968 work *Pastoral Care in Hospitals*, points out that chaplaincy ministry and parochial ministry are both the same and different:

> *Fundamentally of course the work is identical, with its concern for people and their needs; the same shepherding and the same caring. There will be the inevitable limitations of time which both will suffer, but there will be obvious differences. (Autton 1968, p.3)*

At the heart of his model are relationships: the relationship of the chaplain with the hospital community and the relationship of the chaplain with the patient. As Swift (2009, p.46) notes 'Autton's introduction indicates that the priest in hospital is "chaplain rather than clinician and he works not to compete but to complement"'. This working as part of a wider team of healthcare professionals, respecting and understanding the contribution of colleagues and learning to converse in the language of the community marks the transition from being the parish priest in the hospital to becoming part of a new community.

Mark Cobb in his 2004 'contextual model' suggests that chaplains have a distinctive role within the healthcare community in that they not only care for patients and families but also for members of staff, students and all who work within the healthcare organisation. This can render locating the chaplain within the healthcare community ambiguous, as that placement is understood in the context of relationships. Cobb (2004, p.12) writes that chaplains 'may consider themselves advocates of the vulnerable and powerless (staff and patients) or they count themselves as equals among their fellow professionals with a seat at the most important meetings'. In this Cobb highlights one of the challenges for chaplains within the healthcare community: how do chaplains understand and work with questions of power?

Cobb (2004, p.11) goes on to assert that the place of chaplains within healthcare can be described by considering their identity and that identity is made real in the relationships they have with others: 'Chaplains cannot simply go around claiming a particular identity; the communities they relate to and deal with must validate it.' Chaplains cannot construct an identity for themselves without it being understood and accepted by the different communities in which they operate and it is only in relation to these communities that the chaplain's identity has any real meaning.

In his 1971 book *The Hospital – A Place of Truth* Michael Wilson understands that hospitals are communities that are weakened by change and medical advances and chaplains are most effective within those communities when they are themselves. As Swift (2009, p.47) comments: 'For this reason, time and again, the significance of the chaplain is seen to rest in his personal qualities and how he relates to both patients and staff in the hospital.' The chaplain as friend was the image most recognised by patients in Wilson's research. This non-technical generalist, in, but not of, the organisation, who has the personal qualities that makes them a welcome companion on the journey through the hospital is a useful concept to use in designing chaplaincy practice models.

Autton's model also takes into account the distinctive nature of the chaplain's relationship with the patient, which is usually short-lived and must be built and dissolved within days or weeks. These are relationships that are frequently more intense in nature than would be found outside the hospital on a regular basis due to the context in which they are formed and which are further challenged by the limitations imposed by competing demands on the patient's time.

At the heart of Peter Speck's 1988 book *Being There: Pastoral Care in Times of Illness* are pastoral relationships, real encounters with patients, families and staff. Speck describes 'the inter-relatedness of caring' in which he examines the different interfaces of the pastoral situation. The interfaces he describes are between: family and healthcare professionals; family and pastoral carers; pastoral carers and healthcare professionals; and at the point where all three meet is the sick person. Each group may offer a degree of support to the other but may also compete with one another, particularly when roles overlap, to have their own needs recognised. This competitiveness may detract from the ability to care for the sick person and in multi-disciplinary working this is an important insight of which to be aware. The sick person is at the centre of all these relationships and, whilst it is the sick person who is the focus of receiving care, they too may have a part to play in giving; it is by listening to the sick person and allowing them to contribute that their dignity may be maintained or restored.

Education, training and reflection

In order that the chaplain can stand alongside other professionals working within the hospital team, training and reflection are vital elements both in preparation for and in continuing support of a chaplain's hospital ministry. Norman Autton writes 'His position must not be less professional than that of other members of staff, and his science and skill not less marked than those of a surgeon' (Autton 1968, p.1). Until this point theological education and priestly formation were regarded as sufficient preparation to undertake hospital chaplaincy; Autton proposed a more formal, context-specific training. Speaking of the chaplain's ministry, Autton (1968, p.114) declares 'if it is to be really effective, if it is to have any significant meaning for all concerned, then the chaplain must have adequate training and preparation'; he recommended a clinical training within the hospital setting. Autton goes so far as to write 'Without training the hospital chaplain's approach can so easily become irrelevant to the needs of his people – both "healthy" and "sick"' (1968, p.115).

Disciplinary communities, as described in Cobb's model, are bodies that exist to regulate and formalise the particular skills and knowledge needed by members to practise their profession and ensure that members meet and maintain competencies relating to those skills and knowledge. Cobb writes 'Chaplains constitute a disciplinary community in the sense that they do similar work and share common intellectual and practical interests' (2004, p.12). In the USA there is a very well defined body of skills and knowledge in which chaplains are required to demonstrate competence in order to practise – Clinical Pastoral Education. In the UK the picture is less unified with no formalised and universally acknowledged set of competencies required to be able to practise as a healthcare chaplain. The disciplinary community gives identity to the chaplain by describing the set of skills, knowledge and competencies needed in the practice of chaplaincy and this complements those already gained in the formation and training undertaken within the faith community.

Woodward asks the pertinent question of 'where is God' in the move towards healthcare chaplaincy becoming a profession? For him there is too much reliance on a pure business model of what it means to be a professional and an obvious lack of any real grappling with an understanding of a conception of God and how this motivates and influences practice for chaplains. Professionalism for chaplains and the way in which this underpins their practice should be a product of their theological reflection on their vocation to chaplaincy ministry. Folland (2006, p.11) writes: 'His (Woodward's) model offers a theological dimension to complement the skills based approach of secular culture. This raises an obvious but curiously neglected discourse about the location of theology in healthcare.'

Wilson understands the chaplain as both exploratory and experimental in their approach to their role; within this there is a strong imperative to push the boundaries and expand the knowledge base on which chaplaincy models are built. There is an emphasis on the need to examine how chaplaincy works in an ecumenical nature, how lay chaplains and volunteers are used and the possibilities around the development of partnerships in teaching and training. As Folland (2006, p.7) notes: 'Prayer, contemplation, thinking and action are at the centre of Wilson's model and contribute to the development of what we might term today the "reflective practitioner".'

'No pastor can be immune from the effects of the pastoral relationship' (Speck 1988, p.17); in this comment Speck highlights the importance of the pastor being in tune with their own needs, their own limitations and their own vulnerability. Developing within oneself a personal understanding of spirituality, health and illness is essential in helping those who are sick make sense of all that is happening to them; Speck suggests several ways in which this philosophy of life may be developed: establishing a support network to combat feelings of isolation, which can be a danger in smaller chaplaincies where there may only be one chaplain, allows for discussion and feedback – vital in an emotionally and spiritually challenging role; further and continuing education helps to develop new skills and provides a means of meeting with other chaplains in similar situations; and supervision in which different pastoral situations can be analysed and the pastor can explore their own and alternative responses. 'Awareness of our own needs and assuring that we attend to them in an appropriate way will enable us to respect and respond to the person who is ill as they search for meaning in that experience' (Speck 1988, p.25).

The pastoral and priestly nature of chaplaincy ministry

James Woodward, a successor of Wilson's at Queen Elizabeth Hospital in Birmingham, in 2002 developed a service model describing healthcare chaplaincy as 'a ministry at a number of distinct but overlapping and interlocking levels of engagement with the institutions and experiences of disease, healing and health' (Woodward 2002, p.22). Woodward explores how the chaplain operates within these areas of influence by examining the various roles of the chaplain. He examines the chaplain as pastor who works with both groups and individuals within the healthcare setting to assess and respond to emotional and spiritual need, to help make sense of life, death, illness and health within a framework of faith and belief. These pastoral relationships are to support those of faith through times of illness and to enable those of no declared faith to perhaps find new meaning and purpose in the changed circumstance of their lives.

The chaplain as interpreter: in Autton's model one of the elements that distinguished a chaplain from a parish priest visiting in the hospital was learning the language of hospitals. This isn't only the technical medical language used by staff when speaking with each other and, too frequently, with patients, but also the language of experiences and emotions. Some may have religious language that they use, others will have no words to describe what is happening to them and yet others will refer to it only obliquely; the interpreter helps each make sense of what is happening to them by hearing both the spoken and the unspoken word and putting them into a language that the individual can understand.

There is a definite intermediary role for the chaplain, working at different levels within the organisation, in fostering a sense of community within a hospital, enabling supportive relationships and helping to make appropriate links. There are times too when the chaplain may need to be an advocate for a patient, or might be a neutral go-between mediating in a dispute between different parties in the organisation.

Mark Folland (2006, p.11) comments 'The assumption is that we cannot build a healthy hospital community without developing good links with the community who own the hospital.' The chaplain working as a bridge builder encourages the local community to become involved with and take some responsibility for their hospital. Woodward envisaged that by fostering this ownership of the hospital the local community will be a resource that the hospital may draw upon and will at the same time be more empowered to take responsibility for their own health and well-being.

Autton reminds chaplains that the base from which they operate is that of their commissioning from their faith community; chaplains are not free agents but are ordained and authorised ministers working as representatives of their faith community. Chaplains are first and foremost ministers of their faith communities and its rites, rituals and mysteries; a vital element to hold onto when working out models of 'being' chaplaincy in an increasingly secular NHS. 'Involving himself in his people's predicament he is to show them the Christ *already at work* in their midst. By the very fact of his priesthood he is called and set apart by God' (Autton 1968, p.1). For Autton the practice model to be used in hospital ministry is very much that of the priest, but the priest in a very different context to the parish and so operating within a distinctive service model.

> *He is there to give meaning to the very existence of the hospital and the purpose of the lives of those who share its work, attempting to make God more real and more relevant... He is there to interpret what God is all about, and to show what he is doing in and for those who are sick members of his Body. (Autton 1968, p.2)*

As society becomes more secular and the population less churched there is a much greater need for someone to help articulate the language of spirituality, the language around the search for meaning and purpose. And in a society and healthcare setting that is fluid and constantly changing there is a need for someone to make connections, to form links, to bridge gaps; this is a role ideally suited to chaplains, who touch lives at every level of an institution.

Where is God?

Wilson considers that hospitals can teach us to rely on technology as the panacea for all sickness rather than understanding that relationships, with ourselves, our communities and God have a profound effect on our health.

> *The modern hospital is making it more difficult for men to see their delivery from sickness as the work of God: and therefore making it more difficult to respond to the living God, by seducing men to respond to the false god of technology. (Wilson 1971, p.29)*

Wilson (1971, p.44) writes, 'The primary task of the Church is to express in its common life the Truth that sets men free to be fully human.' And in the hospital, which can be a place of fragmentation and conflict, of wholeness and truth, the integrity of the chaplain in being fully human, fully part of the institution and fully part of the Church is vital.

The chaplain, fully part of their faith community, enables the hospital that has become technological and scientific to regain an understanding of illness and health as part of what it means to be human. The chaplain achieves this is by being himself, modelling truth and integrity in all his relationships and holding together the sacred and the secular, sickness and health.

Chaplains operate within healthcare organisations as authorised representatives of their faith communities, sensitive to the breadth of understanding present within their faith communities. In the multi-faith context of contemporary British society not all faith communities have an equivalent role to that of the chaplain, or an organised system for authorising such an individual, therefore new roles are being developed that are analogous to that of the chaplain. The practice of healthcare chaplains is resourced and enhanced from the wide breadth and richness of their faith community tradition. Cobb asserts that, 'For the individual chaplain, being a representative of a faith community means having a rich tradition to draw upon, and this enables a distinctive contribution to healthcare' (2004, p.13).

Hearing, interpreting and responding to the stories of individuals and relating these to the stories of faith communities is part of the unique role that the chaplain fulfils within the healthcare setting. Cobb writes, 'Practical theology is both an academic and community discipline that is grounded by the chaplain in the pastoral context of healthcare'

(2004, p.14). Like Woodward, Cobb understands part of the distinctive role of the chaplain as being an interpreter, enabling individuals to locate their lives and their experiences within the wider context of a faith tradition and ultimately a transcendent reality. The identity of the chaplain as faith group representative and practical theologian is one that is validated by the authorisation and licensing of the chaplain by their faith community, making available to the healthcare organisation the resource of the rich heritage, theological understanding and tradition of that faith community.

Generic chaplaincy

Generic chaplaincy is a model that is well established in countries such as the USA, Germany and Greece and has occasionally been used in British hospitals over the past decade, predominantly to cover on-call duties. Kotva (1998) suggests that the main reasons for the growth in generic chaplaincy in the USA include: the use of clinical pastoral education (CPE) as a way of preparing for healthcare chaplaincy ministry; the multiple roles that a chaplain undertakes; and the fact that chaplains are employed by secular organisations who need to meet the many and diverse spiritual needs of their customers. CPE, Kotva says, was a product of theological liberalism, philosophic pragmatism, psychology and religious existentialism in the 1920s and 1930s and 'is thus rooted in several strains of thought that deprecate theological convictions and denominational allegiance' (1998, p.260). The multiple roles of the chaplain include such areas as alcohol counsellor, marriage therapist and ethicist, and concentrating on these roles prevents the chaplain from focusing on their role as spiritual leader. Finally, the array of different spiritual needs among those who use the healthcare facility means that the chaplain has to be broad-based in their spiritual provision. Kotva writes,

> The combination of these factors implicitly, if not explicitly, discourages chaplains from focusing on the content of their own beliefs and encourages a way of interacting with patients that reflects a (supposedly) more neutral, objective and open minded stance. This de-emphasising of one's own particularity is what I call a generic chaplaincy. (Kotva 1998, p.260)

While CPE is not a common feature in British healthcare, the last two factors are certainly present and, combined with the need to make cost efficiencies, may account for the growth in interest in generic chaplaincy over the past decade. There is a potential concern that taking on a generic way of working could lead to a devaluation of chaplaincy, with chaplains becoming simply facilitators rather than spiritual leads.

There are occasions when acting as a generic chaplain is useful, for example, when representing the chaplaincy on hospital committees it is appropriate to act in a generic manner, being a representative from a faith perspective generally rather than from a specific faith. Chaplains who are allocated wards and departments as their areas of responsibility are able, working generically, to visit everyone in the ward regardless of their faith background and to get to know and support staff. However, in both these situations that person is able to call on the resources of other team members when needed – which in reality is multi-faith chaplaincy.

Whilst there is a degree of general spiritual care that can be provided across faith boundaries and is also appropriate for people of no particular faith, there is a great deal of chaplaincy work that requires a chaplain of a particular faith; it is often not possible for generic chaplains to provide faith-specific rites and rituals. There is the potential that generic chaplaincy could lead to the diminishing of patient choice and satisfaction; patients and families might be upset and distressed if they are visited by a generic chaplain rather than one of their own faith or of their choosing. Engelhardt (1998, p.231) remarks 'patients and their families who expect a brand named chaplain may be puzzled, disturbed or deeply disappointed when they receive the services of a generic'.

It has been suggested by some commentators that if generic chaplaincy practice means that a chaplain puts their own religious convictions to one side for the sake of a pastoral encounter, then it makes a mockery of faith and has an adverse effect on pastoral relationships: Delkeskamp-Hayes writes:

> A partner – in whatever discreet and generous manner – altogether failing to take a stand against anything I say cannot have taken me (or himself) seriously... A truly respectful interchange demands a tolerance that is not restricted to an 'anything goes' kindness. It involves a loving acceptance of me as a person (a creation) across the borderline of right and wrong judgements concerning my actions and beliefs. (Delkeskamp-Hayes 1998, p.293)

Other writers are convinced that because the generic chaplain is coming from a particular faith perspective it is impossible for them to take on a neutral role and that in reality the chaplain is operating with an agenda dictated by their beliefs. Kotva remarks:

> To my mind, the biggest problem with generic, supposedly neutral, hospital chaplaincy is that it isn't neutral at all; rather, a particular perspective is smuggled in and authorised under the guise of something more universal and open minded. (Kotva 1998, p.261)

Generic chaplaincy is currently viewed with suspicion by some sections of British healthcare chaplaincy; there is a sense that the main driver for healthcare managers in promoting generic chaplaincy has more to do with staff cuts and cost saving exercises than exploring ways to meet the diverse demands of service users in a pluralistic society.

Conclusion

There is a crisis in contemporary healthcare; a service that began with the noble intention of providing care, free at the point of delivery, for all finds itself facing unprecedented challenges. A chaplaincy service that is able to respond to the changing context of healthcare and facilitate staff and patients in engaging with the spiritual dimension of health and illness is needed now more than ever.

Chaplains need to be able to locate their identity within the wider healthcare team and describe the benefits of their contribution to patient care and the organisation. Models of healthcare chaplaincy are an invaluable tool in achieving these outcomes by providing a widely accessible description of who chaplains are, what they do, how they do it and why. Models aid healthcare colleagues in understanding and making best use of chaplaincy services as well as providing a framework within which the efficacy of chaplaincy can be measured.

If chaplaincy is to make a contribution in facing the crisis in contemporary healthcare it is essential to develop models that can demonstrate this in ways that are accessible to all stakeholders. Chaplaincy has a rich vein of practice and service models, developed, critiqued, implemented and evaluated over the last half century that can be mined and used in designing and developing robust healthcare chaplaincy models in the future. Without such models chaplaincy services will find it increasingly difficult to evidence their worth to healthcare commissioners and providers and their contribution will not be realised.

CHAPTER 4

Biblical Texts, Chaplaincy and Mental Health Service Users

Anne McCormick

Chaplains are by default interpreters. They bring a set of skills and background information from their religious formation, training and work experiences and seek to adapt and apply themselves as faith practitioners and spiritual advisors in new and very different contexts. They interpret their faith in varied surroundings, trying and sometimes not succeeding in their translation given the structures, and strictures of their environment. They are also interpreters of faith and spiritual matters to their work colleagues providing a lens through which work issues can be looked at from both a spiritual and religious perspective. The work of chaplaincy with patients and service users (a service user is a person using mental health services) is often to help an individual explore how they understand what is happening to them; the changes that are taking place; how individuals redefine themselves in the face of illness and life changing events; and what spiritual and religious resources can be used to gain insight and bring relief in the face of suffering.

When bemused colleagues ask a chaplain what they actually *do*, the phrase, 'spiritual care' does not do justice to the complex, skilled support that a chaplain offers through the unique skill set they bring. They are trained in: understanding world religions and sects; theological and ethical reflection; analysis of the faith texts of world religions; the use of prayer and meditation for reflection and enlightenment and personal discipline; pastoral care situations; and confessional contexts. They come to the role equipped with an understanding of not only the religious but also the spiritual dimensions of a person, and experience communicating with a wide range of individuals and groups of all ages through their former roles, that is, bereavement support, marriage preparation and youth work. These skills complement a person-centred model of care in which attention is paid to all facets of life as important to healing, well-being and wholeness.

In the crucible that is modern healthcare, chaplains need to demonstrate their relevance and value. So often chaplains are seen as the well-meaning amateurs without the necessary professional qualifications that inspire respect within the medical world. It is easy for chaplains to lose confidence in their skills when exercising ministry outside of their faith communities, and when among those who have little knowledge of, or respect for their skills and abilities. In consequence some chaplains gain counselling qualifications in order to demonstrate their abilities in ways that are recognisable by fellow professionals. Research is a key factor in demonstrating the value of the distinctive training undertaken by chaplains as part of their ministerial formation. Our religious traditions have a wealth of experience and resources to offer; centuries of wisdom in nurturing the soul and spirit. Chaplains are therefore challenged to tap into such a reservoir of resources and interpret them afresh in changing times.

Christian chaplains have been trained to pay close attention to the spiritual life and to the discipline of personal devotion. They have also been trained to interpret the Bible and to convey the theology of the Bible through preaching, group and individual study. Acts of worship and daily devotion include passages and phrases from the Bible, and scriptural values are adopted in the quest to become the people of God and to embody the Christ-like life. The ethical and moral values of the Bible are embedded in our culture and have passed into the values of everyday life without direct reference to their origins (e.g. going the extra mile, turning the other cheek, treating others as you yourself would be treated). This chapter explores how chaplains translate into their particular work context the insights they have gained in using the Bible, and demonstrates how modern research, both qualitative and quantitative, can help us to examine that work in more tangible ways.

The research project undertaken (McCormick 2011, unpublished dissertation) sought to discover how Christian chaplains were using the Bible within mental health settings. My own experiences as a mental health chaplain alerted me to the way in which both the context in which I worked and insights from my ministerial experience shaped my personal use of biblical texts and themes. It was apparent that the context of mental health chaplaincy was shaping my engagement with, and interpretation of, biblical texts as in like manner liberation and feminist theologies grew out of a distinct time or setting. Questions emerged such as, 'How do chaplains use the Bible as a healthcare tool?' 'How does the work environment and interaction with service users shape the ways chaplains use or refrain from using the Bible?'.

The research revealed the complex nature of the material involved. Consequently it became clear that investigative questions introduced through discussion and interaction would be far more likely to delve deeper into the experience of chaplains than a questionnaire format. Focus groups would allow insights to be drawn out and developed and enable participants to fully understand what was being asked of them. Chaplains might not be aware of the range of their own practice in this area. There are many subtle ways in which chaplains both use, and take for granted, the Bible: prayer and worship, personal formation, discussions concerning ethical issues, loss and bereavement. Two sessions with a focus group were used, the first session opened up the area under discussion and the second developed the ideas identified in the first. The second session, which was deliberately held after a month had elapsed, was more reflective, drawing upon the participants' heightened awareness. In order to sustain participants' awareness during the intervening weeks a journal was designed to record their use of scripture and capture their reflections, adding value to the group discussion and the research in general (see Appendix).

The group explored questions such as: How did the chaplains consider the efficacy of the Bible in their work? Within the sphere of mental health care was the Bible seen as a useful tool? In a chaplain's ministry how integral was the Bible to his/her practice? How did chaplains integrate that tool in a multi-disciplinary environment alongside colleagues from healthcare backgrounds (i.e. nursing staff, psychiatrists and psychologists)?

Another area of investigation explored whether chaplains use a selective approach when using biblical texts with service users and, if so, what were their criteria? The research sought to elicit this evidence by asking the chaplains which texts and biblical themes they considered too negative, and which beneficial, for use in their context. Participant responses could be verified by the keeping of a research journal and by using supplementary questions within the focus groups. Questions included asking: 'What texts should or should not be used with a suicidal person?', 'What texts should or should not be used for a person dealing with guilt and forgiveness issues?' and 'What types of material or passages have you ever avoided in mental health work and why?' The journal allowed comparison between what people said they were doing and what they were actually doing, thus increasing the reliability of the data and record where there were areas of discrepancy (Silverman 2005, p.215).

The journal simply required a single entry sheet per encounter to ease its use. The entry sheet included four headings: setting, purpose, method and presentation. Each heading had a list of options and chaplains could ring more than one or add their own option. Designing a sheet that was simple to use yet yielded complex information was a challenging exercise. The highly nuanced nature of the subject area necessitated a methodical approach to construct the evidence base. Consideration was given to the general categories that would best reflect practice whilst allowing space for personal comment. The sheet recorded who instigated the use of scripture, the scriptural text or theme used, and also how well the use of scripture was received (see Appendix). It was hoped that by including a variety of contexts, purposes and methods the chaplain might give more consideration to practices they might otherwise overlook.

The research highlighted the changing context and difficulties facing chaplains in this setting. The modern mental health chaplain has referrals to see people whose care is very much on a revolving door basis. Shorter stays, periods of leave from the wards, crisis care at home and supported care in the community create a very different environment for mental health chaplains to navigate. In a multi-cultural Britain the Bible becomes one of several religious texts chaplains are expected to provide for those in their care and in that sense becomes one among many resources. As mental health chaplaincy increasingly defines its role as offering spiritual care to anyone with spiritual needs, the distinctive voices of the Bible may become increasingly muted. In this environment many service users challenge the authoritative position of the Bible and many more have simply not engaged in using the Bible. Contemporary society emphasises the individual, personal journey of self-discovery, such an emphasis encourages the adoption of a self-referential hermeneutic when using sacred texts.

Individuals need ways to express themselves on a spiritual level. The need for a spiritual vocabulary to draw on for good mental health is highlighted by Chaplain Lorna Murray. When Murray discusses the significance of spirituality in pastoral relationships she emphasises the importance of enabling service users to have a spiritual vocabulary, 'The language of spirituality enhances the repertoires of healing vocabularies that we have by transforming and transcending understandings. A vocabulary that includes hope and transcendence, forgiveness and grace will be important in how we author our identity' (Murray 2002, p.33). Chaplains will be fluent in such vocabularies because of their ministerial formation, which is not necessarily normative for the service user, as in some cases concepts of loving relationships are stunted through neglect or terrible childhood experiences.

Material written on the practical use of the Bible in mental health appeared to be very limited. Pattison comments in his helpful overview of the area, 'the fact is that pastoral theologians seem to have almost completely avoided considering the Bible... There is an almost embarrassing silence about the Bible in pastoral care theory' (Pattison 2000, p.106). He suggests that the absence is due to the divergence of biblical and theological studies, and an inability to integrate the new insights of critical biblical scholarship into new theological frameworks. Pattison and others are of the opinion, though not universally held, that the Bible is not overly concerned with pastoral care (Pattison 2000, p.107). Gordon Oliver echoed this sentiment when he wrote, 'The purposes of the Gospel writers and editors in bringing together their stories about the actions and teachings of Jesus were not pastoral but missiological' (Oliver 2006, p.27). Common themes arise in what has been written on this subject: issues of the authority of the text and its inspired nature; the original purpose and context of the text versus a contemporary understanding of the text; and the issue of who mediates the biblical material, the care-giver, receiver or the Holy Spirit. Writers in this area have explored the use of texts for insights into morality, guidance, formation, using the consoling and uplifting nature of certain texts and considering the dangers inherent in using others. American pastoral writers have made significant contributions to the literature and will be discussed here in spite of their differing ministerial context.

The use of the Bible by chaplains, as with many other areas of chaplaincy, has been influenced by changes in the way pastoral care has been viewed. Hiltner writing in the 1940s argued in his work, *Pastoral Counseling* that the priorities of those working in pastoral care should not be comfort, discipline and edification as was generally accepted at that time, but that pastoral care was to do with healing, sustaining and guiding (Hiltner 1949). This clearly influences how the Bible is used; a chaplain would be approaching a biblical text very differently if they were offering edification as distinct from guidance. The idea of using the text as a means of disciplining those who have gone astray from its principles and are consequentially suffering is very different from the idea of choosing biblical principles that will offer sustenance in the face of life's difficulties. If the emphasis is on guidance then the patient becomes one who has a choice in responding to all, or part, of what is offered, and not a passive recipient being enlightened as to what they should or should not believe.

Thurneysen (and neo-Barthians) stand in stark contrast as pastoral practitioners of the European/Reformed school to Anglo-American practitioners and writers (Campbell, Lake, Wilson, Tillich etc.) Thurneysen's approach was very church-centred and viewed pastoral care as an extension of the proclamation of the gospel as carried out in the sermon. Care given to the individual was a proclamation of the gospel, 'dependent on the Word as witnessed to in scripture and tradition' (Campbell 2000, p.80). From this stance the Bible takes a prominent position in patient care as edification and cure.

Thurneysen's work laid foundations for a group of American pastoral theologians for whom scripture is placed at the heart of counselling. A well-known exponent of this approach is Jay Adams, an American professor of practical theology (Adams 1986). Adams presents a challenge to those writing on pastoral care who have moved away from biblical principles and courted psychology and psychiatry. Adams is viewed by many to be anti-psychiatry as he argues for use of scriptural care and that the roots of illness lie in sin. In Adams' pastoral care model the counsellor mediates for the individual the counselling of the Holy Spirit.

Adams' work is very much mission-centred and his priority for pastoral care is for the counsellee to attain a right relationship with God from which all else will follow. His extensive use of scripture seems rather prescriptive (finding verses that can be applied to specific mental health conditions) and those of a more liberal tradition would take issue with a perceived move away from a more individualised, person-centred approach to care. For all the criticism of his challenging approach he has made an important contribution to redressing an overemphasis among chaplains on psychology and counselling over and against theology and the role of religion in pastoral care.

Lake, writing in the 1960s, is interesting as a mental health practitioner who interprets the traits of certain illnesses biblically. He describes certain patients as follows, 'compulsively rigid personalities, defending against inner badness by depressive and obsessional mechanisms, take their key text, "Come ye out from among them and be ye separate"'(Lake 1966, p48). He also offers insights into how some people with mental illness respond to use of the Bible. Lake comments on the belief of paranoid patients that certain texts refer directly to them, or are 'messages'. He identifies a dilemma in distinguishing actual insight from God and symptoms of the condition, and discusses how the word of God is drawn into the service of neurotic and psychotic thinking (Lake 1966, p.48). His work highlights the very real difficulties of reflecting theologically within a mental institution.

The move away from using the Bible as a series of moral lessons is reflected by Ferguson, who states the need to maintain the human face of the Bible and avoid tendencies to use it for, 'haranguing moralism, inhibiting legalism or guilt-producing manipulation.' He purports the view that, 'to some extent the "medium is the message" and the one who ministers with scripture must as far as possible embody its message' (Ferguson 1987, p.128). It is in some senses a freer yet more personally demanding approach.

The literary critical study of the Bible came to the foreground in the 1980s. On the one hand this approach required close attention to the structure of the text; on the other hand it explored the Bible as a great piece of literature, rich in imagery and theme (Alter and Kermode 1989). In the same period Alistair Campbell's book, *Rediscovering Pastoral Care* (Campbell 1986) used the biblical images of the pastor as courageous shepherd, wounded healer and wise fool and founded them on current biblical thinking. He discussed the liturgical role of the Eucharist in bringing to mind the woundedness of Christ to the wounded, and other themes such as journey. In my experience such a link was often made by service users grappling with the pain of their conditions. Campbell believed that the care-giver reading the text and the care-receiver have a mine of imagery to explore in the Bible. The images he chooses are selective and it could be argued that Campbell does not address the overall place and authority of the Bible in pastoral care, however the book seems primarily a work to inspire and enrich the pastoral carer's own understanding of their role in pastoral relationships. I disagree with Pattison's argument that in choosing so few specific images Campbell distorts the view given of the Bible (Pattison 2000, p.123); on the contrary he can inspire readers to look at the enormous potential for theological reflection using modern biblical insight and insights from other works of literature.

Pattinson, writing in the 1990s, used the Bible for its ethical dimension by applying the theme of justice to critique the huge changes that Britain's mental health services were undergoing. He suggests that for those in care who have some knowledge of scripture, pastoral diagnosis can be aided by asking what images and texts the individual finds meaningful (Pattison 2000, p.129; Swinton 2001). Here again there is a shift towards exploring how a patient understands and participates in his or her own diagnosis.

Moves within biblical studies to canonical and reader response approaches (Childs 1984; Watson 1993) gave opportunities for exploring the community and individual engagement with the Bible. This is reflected in a less formal way in pastoral care literature by exploration of themes such as a patient's personal narrative and ownership of story. Rowland and Bennett write, 'As with Practical Theology, so in the tasks of doing New Testament Theology there is an interweaving of the threads of tradition, into the web of one's own experience, so the structures of one's own life affects what makes sense in tradition' (Rowland and Bennett 2006, p.9).

Anderson in *The Bible and Pastoral Practice* turns our attention to the use of narrative perspective in pastoral care; he suggests that 'People make sense of their lives through stories they fashion and cultural narratives into which they are born… If we are defined by our stories then caring for people means listening for stories, not historical facts and symptoms' (Anderson 2005, p.201). We will look at where God's story has touched our story and how individuals can, through pastoral care, 'refashion their life story "through the lens" (Anderson 2005, pp.201–202) of God's story, "in this way God's story through scripture becomes fundamental".

Thus the literature of pastoral studies would suggest the Bible can have a serious contribution to make in an individual's care and in critiquing healthcare practices. Literature from the field of psychiatry would also seem to suggest that reading the Bible can have both positive and negative impacts on some individual's mental health. Fallot's psychiatric research draws our attention to the problems that can arise for those with severe mental health:

The not infrequent religious content of delusions and hallucinations; a sense that the metaphoric nature of spiritual ideation may have a negative impact on symptoms of disorganisation and confusion; the involvement of religious language in self-injury (e.g. taking literally the injunction to pluck out the eye if it offend) or violence to others (e.g. demons seen in another person); and the perceived rigidity of religious beliefs and rituals, rigidity that may worsen symptoms and preclude acceptance treatment recommendations. (Fallot 2001, p.110)

Sometimes service users literally need to be 'liberated from the text'. Other examples of biblical wisdom causing difficulty are mentioned by Pargament. He argues that the biblical idea of submitting to God's will can lead to a fatalistic approach to life and thus to, 'errors of explanation and control in coping, unless some role for causal factors and human agency is differentiated from this general belief' (Pargament 1997, pp.343–344).

On the opposite side a study by Koenig and fellow researchers concludes that use of religion can be positive in healthcare. 'In their study sample of 850 men age 65 years and over and experiencing illness, 20% responded to an open ended question that religion was their primary factor in their coping.' In the list of religious activities undertaken participants gave reading the Bible as a factor (Koenig *et al.* 1992 in James and Wells 2003, p.364). The Mental Health Foundation project report 'Strategies for Living' gives a clear indication of the benefits of reading the Bible among other religious activities, 'Reading the Bible can be a helpful or reassuring activity – for some calming and uplifting – for others providing a source of guidance for coping with life – and a means to feeling happier in themselves and thus better (Faulkner and Layzell 2000, cited in Head 2004, p.84).

The literature appears to support the idea that pastoral care can involve using the Bible as an effective tool, however it can be a double-edged sword and needs to be used in a skilled way. Chaplaincy has something distinctive to offer from the faith traditions in their engagement with foundational faith texts and the theological moral and ethical perspectives that they have gained from that study. The next section considers how this skilled work has been demonstrated through the research.

The research seems to suggest that the Bible is used as a resource to be drawn from selectively and not in its entirety. In my own experience the scriptures available on wards are copies of the Gideon's New Testament and Psalms and not the Old Testament, perhaps with the implied suggestion that certain texts are less suitable, important or accessible. Interestingly the Psalms have many instances of what the Psalmist wishes to happen to God's enemies that are hard to stomach and could be used to fuel paranoia. Most often individuals will turn to the guidance section to find prescriptive texts for their situation or begin at the beginning and try and read as one would a novel. Chaplains in the research considered a great many factors before using religious texts, for example: the service user's cognitive ability at any given time; their ability to concentrate; their presentation of mental illness by connecting seemingly random ideas into a whole; a past history of abuse; self-abuse or suicide attempts; educational ability; and the ability to conceptualise ideas.

Chaplains also had the institutions of church and the health trusts to navigate. In a mental health setting where care is taken to protect acutely ill service users from themselves and protect staff from harm, research participants had developed a cautious approach in their work. Chaplains spoke in the focus groups of how easily what was said could be misinterpreted or internalised, cases where an eye for an eye had been carried out quite literally by service users with a religious fixation. Chaplains in the focus group realised that the Bible may be viewed as an authority among service users, and were cautious in offering it to provide solutions that service users might adopt without careful reflection on their own situation. Readings had to be chosen very carefully; for instance, those who were suicidal might find scriptures about the joys of heaven rather appealing in a negative way. All the chaplains in the research were particularly cautious about using the book of Revelation; one suggested it appealed to some service users precisely because it connected with their own revelations and bizarre hallucinatory experiences.

Sponsoring church bodies appeared not to give much structured support to chaplains or provide their own mental health training for them apart from the early, formative ministerial training. Structures of support that enable reflection on use of the Bible in this area are few. Chaplains involved in the research felt a level of disengagement with their sponsoring churches. Some chaplains appeared to have a lack of involvement in liturgical life in their work setting thus opportunities to use scripture were diminished. Chaplains commented that lectionaries were often unsuitable for this context. In the focus groups some chaplains appeared to have little current, daily engagement with scripture in their own discipline. Often working in lone contexts or multi-faith teams it is easy to see how daily devotion in the workplace might get squeezed. However worship settings were the most recorded context for the use of scripture in the journals and certainly appeared in the focus group to be a key platform for its use.

Chaplains have a balancing act in which there are competing factors at play – factors including how they will contextualise the Bible and how readily they feel supported, confident, willing or able to do that in a mental health setting. Clearly their immediate context is that of healthcare, and a lack of understanding and clarity of their role as spiritual care-givers may be impinging on their use of the Bible. Opportunities for development in their chaplaincy role may also be hampered by a lack of structured support from ecclesiastical sponsors. One participant in the research suggested chaplains had much to share with the wider church, 'I suppose my experience is across situations that are every day for me but when I talk to people who work in the Church they're horrified…so perhaps we've got a role there, we've got another interpretation of what's taught in Scripture…we can take back to the Churches.'

The Chaplains participating in the focus group appeared to use the Bible from a cognitive behavioural therapy perspective, showing different ways of understanding the same situation by using scripture from a more positive angle to counter others or reinterpret the texts that were understood as negative – a chaplain in the research described this process as 'reframing'. It is a common practice in cognitive behavioural therapy to use different techniques to help the service user look at things from different perspectives or viewpoints that can often help them be more positive towards themselves or others. Chaplains helped service users to transform negative stories, for instance, ones in which the service user feels guilt and inadequacy. One chaplain described how the story of the crucifixion had both positives and negatives regarding its use. Service users could sometimes link the idea of Jesus' willing sacrifice to their self-harming behaviours. Around Easter, however, expectations of its use were noted as useful to explore death and loss and new life and hope. Here the chaplains appeared to be more confident in their approaches perhaps because of very familiar texts.

Positive texts chaplains cited included a use of the Psalms to empathise with the depths of despair some service users felt. Psalms 22, 121 and 139 were used to explore the concepts of God's aid and God's loving presence as a comfort. Stories such as the parables were favoured as were stories of God's forgiving, loving nature and constancy. One chaplain in the research describes using the woman caught in adultery passage to affirm Jesus' 'gentleness' in his treatment of individuals.

Chaplains working in the contemporary context of mental health are well versed in the popular uses of meditation for relaxation of anxiety and meditation through mindfulness (Segal, Williams and Teasdale 2002). However it appeared the chaplains in the research were not giving the possibilities of biblical meditation much attention. Endean in his work on the Ignation approach seems to be one of only a few voices extolling the value of utilising such approaches (Endean 2006; James 2006). Anthony de Mello's work book on prayer *Sadhanna* offers examples of how the Bible can be used meditatively (de Mello 1984). Benedictine reflection, used carefully with passages expressing God's love and commitment, can be very helpful in supporting a service user's self-worth and helps develop poor concentration skills through repetition and focus.

Chaplains in the research, as in the literature review, felt they were embodying the Christian story and through that expressing a particular way of life. One chaplain commented:

> *for many people who've had such profound experiences of rejection, whether or not we turn up on time for an appointment and whether we remember the appointment whether we follow through promises that we've made... that kind of thing is an embodiment of... what for me I seek to be about... and maybe an articulation of a Bible passage in my head... whether or not the Bible itself gets used.*

Another described being 'soaked in the Scriptures'.

Participants considered their presence and the values they embodied as an integral part of their work, much in the same ways as described by the school of virtue ethics (Macintyre 1981). Their own identification with their faith narrative informed their responses to service users. They hoped to model a way of living that others could relate to whatever their spirituality.

One striking strand from the research was that service users were by no means passive recipients. One chaplain described a service user who expected her to quote chapter and verse. Service users asked questions about the Bible and its position on ethical issues – issues such as suicide, divorce, sexuality – where they felt themselves condemned by the Bible. Some service users took on the identity of biblical characters. Sometimes chaplains in the research were cautious about the Bible being used by service users to provide solutions without applying proper rigour. Chaplains were often asked to respond quickly to rapidly changing conversations and context. One chaplain in the research reflected, 'there are reasons for putting people into liturgy it's very helpful, it's very useful and therapeutic but it does…rather preclude that sort of thing that we encounter of people…in a sense interrupting the flow and saying look…what about this reading what about that point, I don't think I like that or yes I've been abused can I receive communion?'

Major themes have emerged from the research: contextualisation; exploration of what driving forces lead chaplains to shape biblical material the way they do in their workplace; the very individual working environment of mental healthcare; how the Bible can be understood as a healthcare tool; the importance of service user expectations; service user engagement in shaping chaplain's responses; and the need for specialist training and resourcing of chaplains.

Chaplains reported experiencing feelings of inadequacy in their biblical knowledge, however, spoke with great confidence of using biblical themes and imagery in their work. Chaplains were concerned not to exacerbate a person's symptoms by use of the Bible but were often enthused by the discussions they had with service users when discussing the Bible.

Many considerations come into play when using biblical narrative to explore service users' personal histories. For some individuals their stories of abuse are too difficult to retell and can drag the person back into a negative worldview. These individuals needed to work with the here and now and their present narrative. Some individuals with personality disorders have very ingrained ways of thinking; to change their personal narrative can be extremely difficult, fear-inducing and lengthy work. Yes they can have new stories to inform them and to broaden perspective but I suggest they stand alongside the unchanged stories, which act as scars or semi-healed wounds. Chaplains in the research evidenced skills in navigating complex personal narratives and the ability to use the Bible appropriately in these situations. However, there was a wealth of resources from their own traditions that went untapped perhaps due to their dislocation from their formative environments and lack of resourcing from their sending faith bodies. There is clearly a fine line between the integration of ministry into a new context and the integrity of one's foundations. If mental health chaplains are to 'become all things to all people' (1. Corinthians 9:22, New Revised Standard Version), they need to feel confidence in the support of their faith community. More attention needs to be given by the wider church to enriching the ministry of mental health chaplains and in turn being enriched by their insights. Chaplains not only need to seek out nourishment and support from the wider church, but faith communities need to provide structures and opportunity for that to take place; chaplains provide faith communities with the challenge of how they can facilitate better interpretations of key faith texts that are life giving and not life negating.

In a climate in which chaplains need to justify the distinct contribution they make to the organisations within which they minister, and be more confident in the specialist skills they bring, research into areas that demonstrate those specialisms can only enhance the quality of that spiritual care.

Participant number _____

Copy entry _____

Date _____

Use of scripture initiated by: chaplain/service user/both (please circle)

was the service user response: positive /indifferent/negative (please circle)

Length of encounter with service user/patient _____

Categories   please circle one or more in each column

setting	purpose	method	presentation
worship	bereavement	to illustrate a point	anxiety
music	general guidance	exploring a biblical theme	depression
prayer	ethical guidance	using a biblical image	organic dementia
confession	comfort	interpreting the Bible	bi-polar
discussion	confrontation	allowing the text speak for itself	schizophrenic
group work	relationship with God	other please specify below	suicidal
meditation	life's meaning	....	self-harming
reading	sin and forgiveness		recovering addict
other please specify below	other please specify below		suicidal
....	....		other please specify below
			....

Further comments/thoughts

REFERENCES

Adams, J.E. (1986) *A Theology of Christian Counselling*. Grand Rapids, MI: Zondervan.

Alter, R. and Kermode, F. (eds) (1989) *The Literary Guide to the Bible*. London: Fontana Press.

Anderson, H. (2005) 'The Bible and Pastoral Care.' In P.H. Ballard and S.R. Holmes (2005) *The Bible in Pastoral Practice: Readings in the Place and Function of Scripture in the Church*. London: Darton, Longman and Todd.

Autton, N. (1966) *The Hospital Ministry*. London: Central Board of Finance of the Church of England.

Autton, N. (1968) *Pastoral Care in Hospitals*. London: SPCK.

Baly, M. (1991) *As Miss Nightingale Said…* London: Scutari Press.

Barnett, C. (2001) *The Lost Victory: British Dreams, British Realities. 1945–1950*. London: Pan Macmillan.

Beattie, T. (2007) *The New Atheists: the Twilight of Reason and the War on Religion*. London: Darton, Longman and Todd.

Bleakley, A. (2005) 'Stories as data, data as stories: Making sense of narrative inquiry in clinical education.' *Medical Education 39,* 534–540.

Broyard, A. (1992) *Intoxicated by My Illness: and Other Writings on Life and Death*. New York: Ballantine.

Buber, M. (1944) trans. R. Gregor Smith. *I and Thou*. Edinburgh, UK: T&T Clark.

Campbell, A. (1984) *Moderated Love: A Theology of Pastoral Care*. London: SPCK.

Campbell, A.V. (1986) *Rediscovering Pastoral Care* (second edition). East Kilbride, Scotland: Darton, Longman and Todd.

Campbell, A.V. (2000) 'The Nature of Practical Theology.' In J. Woodward and S. Pattison (eds) *The Blackwell Reader in Pastoral and Practical Theology*. Oxford/Malden, MA: Blackwell.

Carrette, J. and King, R. (2005) *Selling Spirituality*. London: Routledge.

Cassell, E.J. (1991) *The Nature of Suffering and the Goals of Medicine*. Oxford, UK: Oxford University Press.

Charon, R. (2001) 'Narrative medicine: A model for empathy, reflection, profession, and trust.' *Journal of the American Medical Association (JAMA) 286,* 15, 1897–1902.

Charon, R. (2005) 'Narrative medicine: Attention, representation, affiliation.' *Narrative 13,* 3, 261–270.

Charon, R. (2006) *Narrative Medicine: Honoring the Stories of Illness*. Oxford, UK: Oxford University Press.

Charon, R. (2009) 'Narrative medicine as witness for the self-telling body.' *Journal of Applied Communication Research 37,* 2, 118–131.

Child, K. (1965) *Sick Call: A Book on the Pastoral Care of the Physically Ill*. London: SPCK.

Childs, B.S. (1984) *The New Testament as Canon: An Introduction*. London: SCM.

Chochinov, H. (2007) 'Dignity and the essence of medicine: The A, B, C, and D of dignity conserving care.' *British Medical Journal (BMJ) 335,* 184–187.

Cobb, M. (2004) 'The location and identity of chaplains: A contextual model.' *Scottish Journal of Healthcare Chaplaincy 7,* 2, 10–15.

Coulehan, J. (2005) 'Today's professionalism: Engaging the mind but not the heart.' *Academic Medicine 80,* 10, 892–898.

DasGupta, S. (2003) 'Reading bodies, writing bodies: Self-reflection and cultural criticism in a narrative medical curriculum.' *Literature and Medicine 22,* 2, 241–256.

DasGupta, S. (2008) 'The art of medicine: Narrative humility.' *Lancet 37,* 980–981.

De Mello, A. (1984) *Sadhanna: A Way to God, Christian Exercises in Eastern Form.* New York: Doubleday/Image Books.

Delkeskamp-Hayes, C. (1998) 'A Christian for the Christians, a Christian for the Muslims! An attempt at an argumentun ad hominem.' *Christian Bioethics 4,* 3, 284–304.

Department of Health (2009) *Religion or Belief: A Practical Guide for the NHS.* London: Department of Health.

Department of Health (2012) 'The NHS Constitution for England.' Available at: www.dh.gov. uk/prod_consum_dh/groups/dh_digitalassets/@dh/@en/documents/digitalasset/ dh_132958.pdf (accessed 11 February 2015).

Driver, T. (1991) *The Magic of Ritual.* San Francisco, CA: Harper. (Republished 2006 as *Liberating Rites: Understanding the Transformative Power of Ritual.* LLC: BookSurge.)

Endean, P. (2006) 'The Bible in personal formation: A dialogue.' *Contact 150,* 41–43.

Engel, L.G. (1962) *Psychological Development in Health and Disease.* Philadelphia, PA: E.B. Saunders Ltd.

Engelhardt, H.T. (1998) 'Generic chaplaincy: Providing spiritual care in a post-Christian age.' *Christian Bioethics 4,* 3, 231–238.

Fallot, R.D. (2001) 'Spirituality and religion in psychiatric rehabilitation and recovery from mental illness.' *International Review of Psychiatry 13,* 101–115.

Ferguson, D.S. (1987) *Biblical Hermeneutics: An introduction.* London: SCM.

Folland, M. (2006) *A Review of Some Theoretical Models of Healthcare Chaplaincy Service and Practice.* Rotherham: South Yorkshire Strategic Health Authority.

Foucault, M. (1973) *The Birth of the Clinic.* London: Routledge.

Frank, A. (1995) *The Wounded Story Teller: Body, Illness and Ethics.* Chicago, IL: University of Chicago Press.

Frankl, V. (1962) *Man's Search for Meaning.* London: Hodder and Stoughton.

Gordon, T., Kelly, E. and Mitchell, D. (2011) *Spiritual Care for Healthcare Professionals: Reflecting on Clinical Practice.* London: Radcliffe Publishing.

Graham, L.K. (1992) *Care of Persons, Care of Worlds: A Psycho-systems Approach to Pastoral Care and Counselling.* Nashville, TN: Abingdon Press.

Head, J. (2004) 'Please pray for me: The significance of prayer for mental and emotional well being.' The Royal College of Psychiatrists. Available at: www.rcpsych.ac.uk/PDF/ head_8_4_04.pdf (accessed 12 February 2015).

Hiltner, S. (1949) *Pastoral Counseling.* Nashville, TN: Parthenon Press.

Illich, I. (1990) *Limits to Medicine: Medical Nemesis - The Expropriation of Health.* London: Penguin Books.

James, R. (2006) 'The Bible in personal formation: a dialogue.' *Contact 150,* 44–48.

James, A. and Wells, A. (2003) 'Religion and mental health: Towards a cognitive-behavioural framework.' *British Journal of Health and Psychology 8,* 3, 359–376.

Kelly, K.T. (1992) *New Directions in Moral Theology: The Challenge of Being Human.* London: Geoffrey Chapman.

Kitwood, T. and Benson, S. (1995) *The New Culture of Dementia Care.* London: Hawker Publications Ltd.

Kotva, J.J. (1998) 'Hospital chaplaincy as agapeic intervention.' *Christian Bioethics 4,* 3, 257–275.

Kübler-Ross, E. (1997) *The Wheel of Life.* New York: Scribner.

Lake, F. (1966) *Clinical Theology: A Theological and Psychiatric Basis to Clinical and Pastoral Care.* London: Darton, Longman and Todd.

Lewis, C.S. (1942) *The Screwtape Letters.* London: Geoffrey Bles.

McCormick, A. (2011) *In Mental Health Chaplaincy what significant conclusions can be drawn from the Biblical texts Christian Chaplains employ with Service Users,* unpublished dissertation.

McFadyen, A.I. (1990) *The Call to Personhood.* Cambridge: Cambridge University Press.

McGilchrist, I. (2009) *The Master and His Emissary: The Divided Brain and the Making of the Western World.* New Haven, CT and London: Yale University Press.

McSherry, W. (2007) *The Meaning of Spirituality and Spiritual Care Within Nursing and Health Care Practice*. London: Quay Books.

MacIntyre, A.C. (1981) *After Virtue. A Study in Moral Theory*. Notre Dame, IN: University of Notre Dame Press.

Martin, E. (1992) *The Woman in the Body: A Cultural Analysis of Reproduction*. Boston, MA: Beacon Press.

May, W. (1987) 'Care and Covenant or Philanthropy and Contract.' In S. Lammers and A. Verhay (eds) *On Moral Medicine*. Grand Rapids, MI: Eerdmans.

May, W. (1996) *Testing the Covenant: Active Euthanasia and Health Care Reform*. Grand Rapids, MI: Eerdmans.

Meakin, R. and Kirklin, D. (2000) 'Humanities special studies modules: Making better doctors or just happier ones?' *Medical Humanities 26*, 49–50.

Merleau-Ponty, M. (1962) English edn, trans. Colin Smith. *Phenomenology of Perception*. London: Routledge and Kegan Paul.

Montgomery, K. (ed.) (1979) 'Narrative.' In W.T. Reich (ed.) *Encyclopedia of Bioethics*. New York: Macmillan Library Reference.

Mowat, H. (2008) *The Potential for Efficacy of Healthcare Chaplaincy and Spiritual Care Provision in the NHS (UK)*. Aberdeen: Mowat Research Limited.

Murray, L. (2002) 'The significance of the spirituality of the mental health chaplain within the pastoral relationship.' *Contact 138*, 10–35.

NHS Scotland (2009) *Spiritual Care Matters: An Introductory Resource for all NHS Scotland Staff*. Edinburgh, UK: NHS Education for Scotland.

Niebuhr, H.R. (1956) *The Purpose of the Church and its Ministry*. New York: Harper Collins.

Noddings, N. (1989) *Women and Evil*. Berkeley, CA: University of California Press.

Noyce, G. (1989) *The Minister as Moral Counsellor*. Nashville, TN: Abingdon Press.

O'Neill, K. (ed.) (2013) *Patient-Centred Leadership: Rediscovering our Purpose*. London: The King's Fund.

Oliver, G. (2006) 'Jesus and pastoral care: Strangers or friends.' *Contact 150*, 26–30.

Outka, G. (1972) *Agape: An Ethical Analysis*. New Haven, CT: Yale University Press.

Paley, J. (2008) 'Spirituality and nursing: A reductionist approach.' *Nursing Philosophy 9*, 3–18.

Pargament, K. (1997) *The Psychology of Religion and Coping*. New York: Guildford Press.

Pattison, S. (2000) *A Critique of Pastoral Care*. London: SCM Press.

Prickett, S. (2002) *Narrative, Religion and Science: Fundamentalism versus Irony, 1700–1999*. Cambridge: Cambridge University Press.

Ramsey, P. (1970) *The Patient as Person*. New Haven, CT: Yale University Press.

Robinson, M. (2010) *Absence of Mind: the Dispelling of Inwardness from the Modern Myth*. New Haven, CT and London: Yale University Press.

Robinson, S. (2008) *Spirituality, Ethics and Care*. London: Jessica Kingsley Publishers.

Rowland, C. and Bennett, Z. (2006) 'Action is the life of all: The Bible and practical theology.' *Contact 150*, 815.

Royal College of Nursing (2011) *Spirituality in Nursing Care: A Pocket Guide*. London: Royal College of Nursing.

Schein, E.H. (1985) *Organizational Culture and Leadership*. San Francisco, CA: Jossey-Bass.

Schwobel, C. (2006) 'Recovering Human Dignity.' In R.K Soulen and L. Woodhead (eds) *God and Human Dignity*. Grand Rapids, MI: Eerdmans.

Segal, Z.V, Williams, J.M.G. and Teasdale J.P. (2002) *Mindfulness-Based Cognitive Therapy for Depression: A New Approach to Preventing Relapse*. New York: Guilford Press.

Seneca, L.A. *Moral Essays III*. Loeb Classical Library 310.

Shaw, M.C. (1988) *The Paradox of Intention: Reaching the Goal by Giving up the Attempt to Reach It*. Atlanta, GA: Scholars Press.

Shorter, E. (1993) 'The History of the Doctor Patient Relationship.' In W.F. Bynum and R. Porter (eds) *Companion Encyclopedia of the History of Medicine*, vol. 2. London: Routledge.

Silverman, D. (2005) *Doing Qualitative Research: A Practical Handbook* (second edition). London: Thousand Oaks/New Delhi: Sage.

Solomon, M. (2008) 'Epistemological reflections on the art of medicine and narrative medicine.' *Perspectives in Biology and Medicine 51,* 3, 406–417.

South Yorkshire Workforce Development Confederation (2003) 'Caring for the spirit: A strategy for the chaplaincy and spiritual healthcare workforce.' London: South Yorkshire Workforce Development Confederation.

Speck, P. (1988) *Being There: Pastoral Care in Time of Illness.* London: SPCK.

Swift, C. (2001) 'Speaking of the Same Things Differently.' In H. Orchard (ed.) *Spirituality in Health Care Contexts.* London: Jessica Kingsley Publishers,.

Swift, C. (2009) *Hospital Chaplaincy in the 21st Century: The Crisis of Spiritual Care in the NHS.* Farnham, Ashgate Publishing Ltd.

Swinton, J. (2001) *Spirituality and Mental Healthcare: Rediscovering a 'Forgotten' Dimension.* London: Jessica Kingsley Publishers.

Swinton, J. (2006) 'Identity and resistance: Why spiritual care needs "enemies".' *Journal of Clinical Nursing 15,* 7, 918–928.

The Patients' Association (2011) 'We have been listening, have you been learning.' Available at: www.patients-association.com/wp-content/uploads/2014/08/Patient-Stories-2011.pdf, accessed on 1 April 2015.

Thomasa, D.C. (1999) 'The Basis of Medicine and Religion.' In S. Lammers and A. Verhay (eds) *On Moral Medicine.* Grand Rapids, MI: Eerdmans.

VandeCreek, L. and Burton, L. (eds) (2001) *Professional Chaplaincy: Its Role and Importance in Healthcare.* New York: The Healthcare Chaplaincy.

Watson, F. (ed.) (1993) *The Open Text: New Directions for Biblical Studies?* London: SCM.

Weil, S. (1951) *Waiting on God.* London: Routledge and Kegan Paul.

Weil, S. (1952) *Gravity and Grace.* London: Routledge and Kegan Paul.

Whipp, M. (1999) 'A healthy sense of vocation? The state of the vocational ethic in contemporary medical practice.' *Contact 122,* 3–10.

White, G. (2006) *Talking about Spirituality in Health Care Practice.* London: Jessica Kingsley Publishers.

WHO (1998) *Life in the 21st Century: A Vision for All.* Geneva: World Health Organization.

Whorton, B. (2011) *Reflective Caring: Imaginative Listening to Pastoral Experience.* London: SPCK.

Wilson, M. (1971) *The Hospital, a Place of Truth: A Study of the Role of the Hospital Chaplain.* Birmingham, UK: University of Birmingham.

Woodward, J. (2002) 'Health care chaplaincy research for healthcare chaplaincy: A reflection on models.' *Modern Believing 41,* 2, 20-30.

Young, F. (1990) *Face to Face: A Narrative Essay in the Theology of Suffering.* Edinburgh: T&T Clark.

PART 2

Negotiating Spiritual Care in Public

CHAPTER 5

The Value of Spiritual Care

Negotiating Spaces and Practices for
Spiritual Care in the Public Domain

Andrew Todd

Introduction

This chapter will identify spiritual care as a contested practice in
modern healthcare, shaped by the norms of a variety of secularities; and
subject to the critique of different secularist voices; within the wider
context of modern liberal democracies. The chapter will show how
healthcare chaplaincy and the wider spiritual care practice shared with
other healthcare professionals has adapted within such an environment
(out of a history of Christian chaplaincy), developing: new models of
chaplaincy (including multi-faith teams and 'generic' approaches); new
discourses (e.g. those that distinguish between 'spiritual' and 'religious'
care); multi-faith spaces for prayer, worship and reflection; and
frameworks for professionalising public practice. Such developments
will be set within their political context, for example in relation to
norms of 'patient choice', and of respect for diversity and the provision
of equal opportunity.

The chapter is concerned, therefore, with exploring how the public
value of healthcare chaplaincy is negotiated. This will be examined
through the use of an original analogy, drawn from the world of
international relations, that compares security responses to 'threat', with
'secular' responses to 'risk'. The chapter also reflects on such responses
as a negotiation of the contemporary secular sacred (Cf. Lynch 2012;
Pattison forthcoming), providing particular examples. The chapter
concludes that chaplaincy's distinctive contribution to healthcare lies

in its adaptable and creative negotiation of space to continue offering spiritual, religious and pastoral care as a public service.

This paves the way for other chapters in this section. Chapter 6 by Layla Welford explores the detail of the current UK legal and policy framework for healthcare chaplaincy, indicating inadequacies currently needing to be addressed. Chapter 7 by Mirabai Galashan is a robust consideration of the further adaptation necessary for healthcare chaplaincy to fully respond to the increasing diversity and decentralisation of faiths and beliefs in both the UK and the USA. And Chapter 8 by Debbie Hodge offers insight into a particular approach to evaluating practice in the context of human encounters between chaplains, patients, carers and staff. This emerges, within the current political context, from a dialogue between chaplaincy and nursing theory and practice, and from shared reflection with chaplains.

Secularity and secularisms shaping chaplaincy

The chapter makes an assumption, indicated earlier, that the public value of any kind of chaplaincy (and indeed of other aspects of religion/spirituality) is shaped by the secularity of the context, at both national and more local levels. Such secularities are shaped in turn by the competing secularisms that bid to determine the rules, norms and boundaries of secular public life (of the prevailing secularity).

This assumption is justified first by a working definition that holds the secularity of a particular context to be defined by the way in which the norms of public life, including policy and legislation, order or constrain religion in the public domain. Such norms would include those of liberal democracies, focused in espoused values such as tolerance and fairness. They would also include an assumption that the well-being of society and its public life is determined by the state of the 'Economy' (reified as part of the modern social imaginary; see Taylor 2004, Chapter 5). Further, secularity is determined by a range of norms to do with rights, freedoms and their limitations, including: human rights; understandings of equal opportunity and diversity; security (e.g. the prevention of 'extremism'); and norms of social integration or cohesion (involving shared, or national values).

It is important to note, therefore, that secularity is only one aspect of the way the public domain is established. It is located within wider frameworks of public norms and reasoning, which do not only have to do with religion. Secularity is therefore one aspect of modernity. Also of importance is the understanding that secularity is not simply about a secular/religious *divide*. Rather, secularity concerns the interaction of religion within secular domains. It is therefore about the kind of boundaries drawn around religion. There are those secularists (to be discussed further below) who would wish there to be a distinct, or impermeable, boundary around 'religion' such that it is only able to operate as a 'private' domain. But this is not a political reality within any actual liberal democracy. Even in France, which has a strong principle of *laïcité*, of separation between church and state, religion still operates in the public domain. This is exemplified by the existence of chaplains of different faiths in French hospitals, prisons and the military. The boundaries drawn around religion in liberal democracies are therefore permeable, to different degrees, allowing for different degrees of interaction of religion and public life, and the participation of religion in civil society.

Those representing different secularisms bid to render such boundaries more or less permeable. At the hard end of the secularist spectrum (as indicated above) some will lobby for religion to be regarded only as a private activity, in particular seeking to reduce, or eradicate public funding for activities such as chaplaincy.

Another secularist position that seeks to manage or control religion is predicated on the view that it is problematic. This may be argued on the grounds that religion is 'irrational', and therefore not able to participate straightforwardly in public reasoning. It may be that the 'problem' is identified as religion's tendency to proselytise. Or it may be that religion is regarded as dangerous, because it promotes, or gives rise to, 'extremism' that may lead, in turn, to violence and terrorism.

In some sense the mirror image of the previous secularism is the view of religion as resource. Faith communities may be appealed to as a source of useful values in the search for social integration. They may also be co-opted as agents of monitoring or control. This has been one aspect of the experience of Muslim prison chaplains in England and Wales, as they have been involved by government in the Prevent Strategy, and involved in the prevention of 'extremism' (see Todd 2013).

'Softer' secularisms, that establish positively the public role of religion would include those that enable religion and belief to be seen as right. The European Convention on Human Rights establishes the right of the individual to manifest and change their beliefs.[1] And in the UK the 2010 Equality Act establishes religion and belief as one of the 'protected characteristics'. This sits alongside a historic British 'secularism', that of 'establishment', which gives rise to a set of inherited norms, by which the interaction of church and state is enabled. The latter two secularisms in particular illustrate that a 'secularism', an ideological position about religion and public life, represents a model of the interaction of religion and belief, and the state.

In order to further justify the hypothesis that chaplaincy is shaped by secularity and secularisms, it is worth establishing an overview of the way this works in healthcare. The dimensions of the secularity of the NHS are various. They include the integrity of healthcare as a social and professional domain (on the secularity of 'institutional domains', see Wohlrab-Sahra and Burchardt 2012). Religion is shaped within that domain in order to safeguard the identity of healthcare as a professional arena, as religious practices are conformed to the driving models of healthcare practice. For example, spiritual care in a number of documents developed by UK healthcare chaplains (see e.g. NHS Education Scotland 2008), constructs chaplaincy activity as 'assessment' of 'spiritual need', leading to appropriate 'intervention'. In some sense, this 'medicalises' the traditional chaplaincy practice of pastoral care.

Given the 'economism' of the public sector, including its impact on health (seen as commodification and the growth of seeing the patient as 'consumer' of healthcare), religion in health is constrained by cost–benefit analysis (and must find its place in the 'market'). One aspect of this dynamic is the argument for and against an 'outcomes'-based approach to chaplaincy and spiritual care. This is a live debate on both sides of the Atlantic (see, e.g. Handzo *et al.* 2014). There is a nexus here that connects a focus on evidence-based practice (with a corresponding emphasis on developing a research base) and economic value.

Ethical norms also contribute to the ordering of religion in health, notably those that emphasise autonomy, rational choice and 'patient experience'. For instance, established norms of healthcare ethics, such as autonomy, justice, non-maleficence and beneficence (Beauchamp and Childress 1994), may be seen to act as a mediating language, providing a context into which wider, less health-specific ethical norms (including faith-based frameworks) are translated.

The particular effect of a framework of human rights, respect for diversity and a public duty to promote equal opportunity on healthcare chaplaincy will be discussed later. But its effect is significant, arguably giving rise to a new discourse of 'spiritual care'. Alongside this political agenda, and also shaping the work of chaplains (as well as all other health professionals) is the political concern to protect 'vulnerable' people. This includes protecting people against the more 'dangerous' effects of religion, resulting in a public suspicion of (and possibly taboo against) proselytisation, as well as concern to protect people from 'extremism'.[2]

Different voices, representing a variety of secularisms (in the sense outlined previously), bid to shape the interaction between chaplaincy and the different dimensions of the secularity of public healthcare. At the harder end of the secularist spectrum, the National Secular Society has conducted campaigns in both England and Wales, lobbying for the redirection of public funding from chaplaincy to other areas of healthcare (see National Secular Society n.d.). A variety of parties include within their role that of the management and/or governance of chaplaincy. These would include the Diversity Lead in an NHS Trust, and a variety of managers and trustees with responsibility for working with policies on spiritual care. Alongside these, chaplains' roles include that of promoting an appropriate secular framework that enables their engagement as faith practitioners within a public domain. Thus, for example, in both the UK and the USA chaplains have developed frameworks for the registration and accreditation of chaplains, accompanied by published professional standards and expectations about what makes a chaplain fit and safe to practise.[3]

What kind of negotiation?

The above picture of the secularity of healthcare sets the context in which chaplains negotiate their identity, and provides first examples of chaplains legitimating their practice. This section of the chapter addresses the question of the nature of such negotiation, by way of an analogy.

This arises out of the concept, from the field of international relations (IR), of 'securitisation', which involves constructing a situation primarily in terms of security – especially as an emergency, crisis, risk, or threat. This concept was developed within the 'Copenhagen School' (e.g. Buzan *et al.* 1998). In IR the concept is deployed to create the possibility of rule-breaking. For example, if securitisation leads to the identification of a state as 'failing' or 'failed', then international action may be taken that infringes the sovereignty of that state. In contemporary events, Syria has been both 'securitised', as intervention in relation to the Syrian civil war was contemplated by governments in the summer of 2013, including those of the USA and UK, and potentially desecuritised, as the possibility was discussed in summer 2014 of cooperation between international forces and President Assad, in order to tackle a different security threat posed by those calling themselves 'Islamic State'. Language adopted in such situations, including that of the 'failed state', represents the 'grammar of security', which gives rise in turn to the securitisation 'plot' that justifies international action to counter the 'threat', including the possibility of military action.

By analogy, this chapter proposes a new way of understanding the word 'secularisation', as constructing a situation as risk, or threat, to the secularity of a context. As in security-driven parallel situations, the risk that the secularity of a country, or organisation, may be compromised gives rise to elements of 'grammar' and 'plot', justifying intervention and constraint. The aim of such action is to reduce the risk and, in the extreme, to neutralise the 'threat', to the prevailing secularity. This might involve constructing and deploying norms predicated on rationalism, tolerance or fairness; and more extreme measures, including removing public funding and accreditation. A prominent contemporary example of such secularisation would be the government response to certain schools in Birmingham in 2014, following the so-called 'Trojan Horse plot'. As one aspect of the situation, the actions of certain governors were constructed as having the aim of 'Islamification' of schools, likely to promote 'extremism'. This provided a narrative of governors' actions as a threat to the secularity of the schools. It was clear from public debate reported in the media that this was not the only way in which the situation was perceived by those involved. But it appeared to have the effect of justifying unusual intervention by Ofsted and the reduction of 'risk' by placing certain schools in 'special measures'. The narrative contributed therefore to constraining the role of the schools' governing bodies and the perceived influence of religion in state schools.

The suggestion here is that there are different possible responses to being secularised in this way that may be adopted by religious actors. One response might be termed 'religionisation' (with apologies to those who favour plain English!) – constructing public intervention into the religious domain as, in turn, a risk, or threat, to theological purity. For example, in the wake of same-sex marriages being made legal in England and Wales, some churches have responded by re-emphasising a different perspective on marriage (that it is only between a man and a woman) and indicating that state law will not alter church marriage discipline and practice. This is a response involving a degree of separation from the public domain.

An alternative response involves engagement with the public domain – (re)-negotiating a role for religion in the public space. Once again IR provides an analogy, or model, in what is known as a 'positive security' approach (Hoogensen Gjorv 2012). Such approaches characteristically have the aim of bringing different parties to the table. These parties include those, such as insurgents, who have been labelled as 'dangerous actors'. The dialogical approach therefore has the effect of reversing the 'securitisation' of these actors. Those involved work with underpinning values, including those in play at local level; and are thus contextual. And they see security as a means to a greater end, broadly the re-establishment of peace and justice, rather than as simply protection from risk.

By analogy, as will be shown from particular examples, effective engagement by chaplains and others with secular constraints, may be seen as a 'positive secular' approach. By becoming involved, and involving others, in dialogue amongst different parties (including apparently 'dangerous' religious actors – those perceived as threat to the secular); by using a contextual approach that acknowledges local values and practices; and by proceeding, at least implicitly, on the assumption that secularity can enable wider aims (such as good health and healthcare), chaplains have successfully negotiated not only a presence in public life, but an active role in civil society.

The other dimension of such positive engagement in the secular arena, identified by this chapter is working with the contemporary secular sacred. By 'sacred', in this context, is meant transcendent norms around which a social group orientates itself, through shared narratives and ritual that contribute to social ordering (see Lynch, 2012). Such norms may further be characterised as 'sacralities' – aspects of the sacred (see Pattison, forthcoming). Sacralities are not fixed for all time, and may wax and wane in importance over time and in different contexts. For example, Lynch discusses the change and interaction of the sacred values of priestly authority and the child, in relation to abuse in residential homes in Ireland in the 20th century (2012, Chapter 3). Further, contemporary sacred norms may be religious or secular, or a complex mixture of the two.

In relation to the earlier discussion of responses to being secularised: that of 'religionisation', or separation between religious and secular values, might be characterised as protecting the purity of the religious sacred;

while engagement with secular values might be regarded as working with, and sometimes establishing, the secular sacred. The hypothesis explored in this chapter is that chaplains, and healthcare chaplains in particular, have become actors in local negotiations of secularity. They engage with the secular sacred, contributing symbolic capital (Bourdieu 1986) (such as religious ethos, humanitarian presence, a moral tradition, particular understandings of health, education, economic well-being), through local practices (pastoral care, ritual, organisational involvement, offering peopled spaces). In the process chaplaincy becomes a public activity and presence, and chaplains and their religious traditions are (re)valued as such.[4]

Continuing to develop the hypothesis in terms generated by the discussion of secularity and secularisms earlier in the chapter, chaplaincy takes the opportunity of softer secularisms to participate in the public secular. This engagement is local, contextual, multi-actor and positive – exploring how the prevailing secularity can enable religious participation in public matters (such as healthcare). This involves negotiating out of the trap of being 'secularised'; discovering, and participating in, the public sacred (in symbolic ways that may attract financial investment); and relocating religious 'sacralities' as they interact with secular values. In exploring whether and how this actually happens in practice, the researcher might be advised to follow the money! Significant clues to the public valuing of chaplaincy and its symbolic capital lie in the financial capital that particular aspects of chaplaincy attract. A key question is: What aspects of symbolic work attract public money? The answer to this casts light on how chaplains' symbolic work contributes to particular elements of the public sacred (or transcendent social norms).

Multi-faith spaces act as a particular example of a continuing process of valuing religion in public places (including universities, hospitals, prisons, shopping centres, airports and others). Significant investment in such spaces is evident from the Manchester University research project investigating them (School of Environment and Development n.d.). The development of multi-faith spaces is often justified in relation to a significant aspect of the public secular sacred – human rights, equal opportunity and respect for diversity. They provide for individual freedom to manifest one's belief, and allow for the management and promotion of diversity and social integration.[5] At the same time, and in interaction with the rights discourse, religion or spirituality appears to act as a resource, offering people the opportunity to be apart from the main business of the organisation in which the space is located, offering stillness;[6] or 'safe' space (see Todd and Tipton 2011). Thus some of the distinctive spatial and ritual practices of different faith traditions are valued in new ways as they are held within a shared secular human rights framework. This involves the co-existence and renegotiation of diverse religious sacralities, and gives rise to new language (centred on the very term, 'multi-faith') and shared practice.

Healthcare examples of negotiating the secular sacred

The chapter next seeks to establish that the hypothesis discussed previously is grounded in, and evidenced by, the reality of healthcare chaplaincy. In each case, the driving secular norm is identified, along with the particular area of organisational life in which the relevant negotiation takes place. The way in which chaplaincy has responded is discussed, together with the tensions or questions that remain.

Example 1: Cost–benefit analysis

Reference was made earlier to the impact of 'economism' on healthcare (seen as commodification and the growth of the patient as 'consumer' of healthcare). The particular secular sacred at work here is cost–benefit analysis – against the wider narrative of the 'market', healthcare provision must be efficient, offer value for money and be competitive. Provision of spiritual care and chaplaincy must in some sense conform to these norms in the negotiation of healthcare budgets, in order to ensure continued public financial resourcing.[7]

This gives rise to one response, also referred to earlier, that chaplaincy and spiritual care should adopt an 'outcomes'-based approach to chaplaincy and spiritual care (see, e.g. Handzo *et al.* 2014). Such an approach, not universally accepted by chaplains, connects a focus on evidence-based practice (with a corresponding emphasis on developing a research base) and economic value. This was also seen in the encouragement given to chaplains in the UK to develop a 'minimum data-set'. This was part of the 'Caring for the spirit' project, designed to support the development of healthcare chaplaincy in the UK, led initially by the South Yorkshire Workforce Development Confederation (2003). In the project's proposal for a minimum data-set for spiritual care, the rationale for the development includes, alongside the benefits for good practice, the argument that the data should be monitored: 'To establish best use of resources'; and 'To provide value for money' (South Yorkshire Workforce Development Confederation 2004, p.2). The proposal encourages the quantification and collection of data on all manner of chaplaincy activities, including encounters, call-outs, referrals and a range of specific duties. Such data have been collected by chaplaincy departments (although not all) and used by at least some to justify funding for the department.

Without doubt, the move to collecting data about chaplaincy activity has enabled conversations between chaplains and others, not least their managers, about the value of chaplaincy and, for example, the need to have a particular number of chaplaincy hours for a particular-sized unit. Arguably the central remaining tension for chaplains is the challenge of quantifying pastoral care. In historic (and continuing) understandings of chaplaincy rooted in Christian theology, it has been characterised as a 'ministry of presence', or as 'incarnational'. Seeing chaplaincy instead as numbers of encounters, significantly revalues the practice, and indeed the justification for chaplains engaging in their traditional activity of 'loitering with intent'! A further temptation of the trend towards quantification and the demonstration of value for money might also be to over-emphasise evidently beneficial services (e.g. end-of-life care).

Example 2: Models of healthcare

In the second example, the driving norm at work is the model of multi-specialist medicine, realised in practice as the workings of the multi-disciplinary team (MDT). Chaplaincy has had an ambiguous relationship with MDTs, which signals ambivalence around whether chaplains are healthcare professionals (on the part of chaplains themselves, as well as others involved in healthcare). But a number of leading chaplains and chaplaincy organisations have been involved in negotiating a professional identity in recent years (see Swift 2014). And the word 'professionalisation' has been significant within the development of chaplaincy on both sides of the Atlantic.[8] The development of a professional framework for spiritual care by NHS Education Scotland pioneered a model that has influenced practice throughout the UK. This framework included a letter from the Chief Executive of the Scottish Government Health Department, standards, the published capabilities and competences referred to earlier (NHS Education Scotland 2008), the development of a funded postgraduate training programme and other resources.[9] The framework as a whole has consolidated the resourcing of chaplaincy in NHS Scotland, including resources for training and professional development.

Another area of negotiation has been around chaplains' access to patients' notes. This is discussed by Layla Welford in Chapter 6. The most significant point here is the ruling of the Information Commissioner following the Data Protection Act 1998 (DPA), that chaplains should not have access to notes without the explicit consent of patients, because the work of chaplains was not included within the definition of 'medical purposes'. Nor did the definition of 'health professional' in the DPA include healthcare chaplains. This issue has not been resolved and local practice varies considerably.

What these cases illustrate is that chaplains are involved in a renegotiation of their professional identity that would in some ways bring them into line with the dominant model of multi-specialism healthcare. The benefit is that it allows chaplains to have a voice in the midst of multi-specialism healthcare. The risk, identified by chaplains themselves, is the potential loss of a role that is distinct from the specialist approach, and which seeks to focus on the human (in a person-centred way) and to make connections across domains – between healthcare specialisms; and between patients (and their life-world) and healthcare professionals (and their language and culture). Once again, a particular process of revaluing chaplaincy both enables and constrains participation in healthcare and the distinctive contribution of chaplaincy.

Example 3: The rights discourse

This example focuses on the contemporary sacralities of human rights, equal opportunity and respect for diversity. The conundrum is how chaplaincy in healthcare (or indeed any public institution) can be provided by faith-specific practitioners for those of diverse faiths and for those of no espoused faith. This is explored further in Chapter 7.

In the face of changing patterns of religious affiliation, public suspicion of proselytisation and hard secularist lobbying that public money should not resource faith-specific services (see previously on the National Secular Society), chaplaincy has needed to demonstrate its engagement with diversity. No longer does an Anglican-dominated historic model of openness to all, but working from a faith-specific model of care, have sufficient political currency to justify public chaplaincy provision. The nature and extent of adaptation has varied in different public settings (see Todd 2011), and has included the development of closer cooperation between Christian denominations and churches, and of multi-faith teams. It has also included the development of 'generic' approaches to chaplaincy practice, although the meaning of the term remains highly contested, especially because at issue is the interaction and boundaries between faith-specific practice and a practice that is responsive to need, and offered on the terms of the service user.

That this is a significant issue in healthcare is demonstrated by the attention paid to equality issues in the development of guidelines for healthcare chaplaincy in England during 2014. The introduction to the draft guidelines argues that:

> The changing nature of communities in England means that chaplains respond to calls of increasing complexity. The diversity of religions, beliefs and cultures within the population has grown and the need for chaplaincy departments to advise providers about equality and access has increased. In addition to religious needs chaplaincy managers must consider how best to determine and deliver spiritual care to those whose beliefs are not religious in nature. In doing this, equality legislation, the NHS Charter and human rights obligations are of vital importance, but critically the experiences of patients, and carers is enhanced by ensuring either religious or non-religious pastoral support is available. In order to put patients first the NHS in England seeks to understand the rich variety of beliefs and values of the population in its care. Chaplains are an essential resource for achieving the ambition to provide high quality care for all and promote the protected characteristics of both religion and belief. It is important to note that chaplains are not alone in providing pastoral or spiritual care and the nursing profession has a long established role in supporting the spiritual well-being of patients. (NHS England 2015, p.7)

This aspect of the case for the future resourcing of chaplaincy is aligned with both NHS England's aim of promoting equality and reducing health inequalities (NHS England 2013), and the 2010 Equality Act.

The major response in healthcare to these issues, on the part of chaplains, nurses and others, has been to develop a new language of 'spiritual care', and to make a distinction between this and 'religious care'. Thus a typical statement holds that: 'Spiritual Care is person centred care which seeks to help people (re)discover hope, resilience and inner strength in times of illness, injury, transition and loss'

(NHS Education Scotland n.d.) A further statement elucidates the relationship between spiritual and religious care:

> *Spiritual care is usually given in a one-to-one relationship, is completely person-centred and makes no assumptions about personal conviction or life orientation. Religious care is given in the context of the shared religious beliefs, values, liturgies and lifestyle of a faith community. Spiritual care is not necessarily religious. Religious care at its best, should always be spiritual. (Scottish Executive Health Department HDL 2002, p.76)*

Spiritual care is something offered to all, whereas religious care is offered to those whose spirituality is lived out in religious ways. The underlying assumption is that all people are spiritual, but only some are religious.

The language represents a significant revaluing of chaplaincy practice. And it seems in practice to provide a publically acceptable discourse that enables chaplains to go on offering person-centred pastoral care, which has been their historic strength, in cooperation with other healthcare practitioners. It also provides a theoretical underpinning for conversations about spiritual need, referred to in relation to the professionalisation of chaplaincy in example 2. Here too, however, there are tensions. There remains a question about whether 'spiritual care', together with the underlying concept of 'spirituality', forms a sufficiently robust theoretical construct to underpin practice.

This may be compounded by the difficulty of achieving clarity about the terms 'spiritual' and 'religious'. In a recent survey by YouGov and Lancaster University (YouGov n.d.), roughly equal numbers (around 10% of respondents in each case) described themselves as a religious person, a spiritual person or both spiritual and religious. But 51 per cent ticked, 'I would not describe myself, or my values and beliefs, as spiritual or religious'. This is juxtaposed with the nearly 60 per cent of the population who identified themselves as Christian in the 2011 census. Across different polls there is no consistent correlation between identification with being religious, or spiritual, and particular religious or social affiliations.

So the language of 'spiritual care' provides a narrative that contributes to the public legitimacy of chaplaincy, as a professional body that contributes to the inclusion of diversity within healthcare. It creates space for chaplains to go on responding to the needs and concerns of patients, carers and staff, whatever their beliefs. But it may disguise the fact that chaplains are good at working with a range of action-driving narratives and beliefs in part because they thoroughly inhabit their own belief community and tradition – their openness grows out of their being religious.

Example 4: Compassion and human dignity

Compassion has come to have a renewed normative value within healthcare in the UK. In part this is because of its inclusion as one of the primary values of healthcare in the current NHS Constitution (NHS n.d.), alongside 'respect and dignity'. But additional impetus has been provided by the development of 'Compassion in Practice' as a nursing vision and strategy in late 2012 (NHS England n.d.), reinforced by the publication of the Francis report[10] on the Mid Staffordshire NHS Foundation Trust in February 2013. The emphasis on compassionate care appears to be a response to a strong feeling that healthcare practice had, in certain prominent cases, failed to be in keeping with respect for human dignity.

Chaplains, as traditional exponents of compassionate pastoral care, have responded to these wider NHS developments. At a workshop on the 'Future of Chaplaincy' on Tuesday 29 October 2013 at St Marylebone Church, London, organised by Hospital/Health Care Chaplaincy (part of the Mission and Public Affairs Division of the Archbishops' Council) Chris Swift identified 'Compassion in Practice' as one of the significant aspects of the contemporary NHS shaping chaplaincy; and highlighted its significance for the development of new guidelines for healthcare chaplaincy in England.[11] This is reflected in the wording of the 2015 guidelines, including the following statement: 'Compassion should inform chaplaincy practice and is a key outcome of the patient's experience of the service being provided' (NHS England 2015, p.10). Chaplaincy is thus revoicing its competency to provide safe compassionate pastoral care against the background of wider NHS developments, but as part of the negotiation of a new organisational framework for chaplaincy in the NHS in England. In this case, NHS concerns about healthcare practice provide the opportunity for chaplaincy to reassert an historic strength, as an asset for the NHS, offering symbolic capital in a time of public scrutiny.

The dynamics of negotiation and alignment

The earlier four examples illustrate different ways in which healthcare chaplaincy has engaged with the contemporary secular sacred, the norms at work in healthcare, adapting and re-presenting their work and identity. But what are the dynamics of negotiation and alignment at work? An analysis of these and other examples, suggests two particular dimensions, or axes. The first of these is the alignment of chaplaincy with models of healthcare, with outcomes ranging from chaplaincy locating close to 'mainstream' models, to chaplaincy presenting as more 'alternative'. The second dimension is about how faith practices are adapted within healthcare, with a range from straightforward accommodation of existing practices, to adaptation and innovation.

Figure 5.1 offers a diagram that locates different choices made by chaplaincy against the two axes.

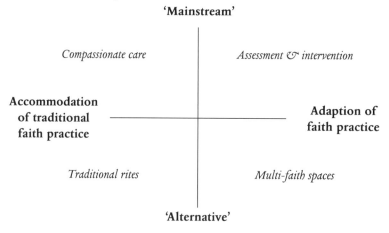

Alignment with models of healthcare
'Mainstream'

Compassionate care   *Assessment & intervention*

**Accommodation
of traditional
faith practice**   **Adaption of
faith practice**

Traditional rites   *Multi-faith spaces*

'Alternative'

Figure 5.1 Alignment with models of healthcare

By way of illustration, this chapter suggests that example 4 from earlier, chaplaincy's response to the NHS's re-emphasis of compassionate care, has provided the opportunity for chaplaincy to align their traditional model of pastoral care (albeit seen today in multi-faith forms) with a mainstream approach to healthcare; whereas the evolution of professional models of spiritual care, constructed as assessment and intervention, while aligning chaplaincy with mainstream models of healthcare, requires rather more adaptation of chaplaincy practice.

In the lower two quadrants of the diagram, traditional rites (including funerals and other end-of-life rites, Friday prayers for Muslims, communion for Christian patients, etc.) are both 'alternative' to more medical practices, and are of value without significant adaptation. But multi-faith spaces, while also 'alternative' have given rise both to the adaptation of traditional approaches to worship and prayer space, and to innovative ritual approaches that respond to a greater diversity of spiritualities.

It could be argued, therefore, that chaplaincy sometimes works in dialogical, alignment with the public sacred – establishing secular models of healthcare; but at other times will embody an alternative (balancing, mitigating or critical) approach to the public sacred – modifying the secular norms of healthcare. In both cases, chaplaincy can contribute a distinctive religious, or spiritual, approach to the secular, by offering the riches of particular faith traditions, or by discovering new practices through adaptation.

In some areas of practice different dimensions are in play at once. Where chaplains are involved in offering mindfulness practice (which is a wider phenomenon than just being associated with chaplaincy), they may find themselves offering something that is an 'alternative' approach to health, but which has also come to be regarded as a mainstream healthcare intervention justified by empirical physiological research.[12] At the same time, mindfulness is rooted in traditional Buddhist (and other faiths') meditative practice, and has been adapted as a practice independent of particular faiths.

Conclusion

The argument of this chapter is that the previous examples demonstrate that healthcare chaplaincy has evolved and developed through positive engagement with different dimensions of the secularity of healthcare in the public domain. The resulting negotiation between a range of chaplains and chaplaincy bodies, on the one hand, and public healthcare organisations, on the other, may be characterised as working with the secular sacred. That sacred includes norms, or sacralities, relating to such areas as cost–benefit analysis, multi-specialism models of healthcare, the human rights discourse and compassion in relation to human dignity. The outcomes of negotiation have included a developing framework for chaplaincy, which has justified continued public resourcing, and has created an organisational space in which chaplains have gone on providing person-centred care for patients, carers and staff. Far from being 'secularised', chaplaincy has discovered ways of contributing a faith dimension to the development of contemporary public healthcare.

In one sense, the distinctive contribution of chaplaincy to healthcare in recent history has therefore been its adaptability and contextuality. The dynamics between alignment with mainstream modes of healthcare and being an 'alternative' resource, and between offering the riches of established faith practices and evolving new practices, illustrate the creativity and resourcefulness of contemporary chaplaincy and spiritual care. However, to place adaptability as the primary distinctive contribution that chaplains make would be to see the situation upside-down. A better perspective would identify chaplaincy's engagement with the secular as a means to an end, that of contributing to contemporary healthcare; by continuing to offer high quality spiritual, religious and pastoral care, as part of a holistic approach to health. This is the true distinctive role of healthcare chaplaincy, which is both rooted in historic traditions of faith, and responsive to an increasing diversity of belief and the changing needs of those who are involved in public healthcare as users or as deliverers.

Notes

1. The most significant article of the Convention is Article 9 (freedom of thought, conscience and religion), but other articles are also significant, including: Article 8 (right to respect for private and family life); Article 13 (right to an effective remedy); and Article 14 (prohibition of discrimination).
2. The latter has given rise, in part, to each NHS Trust and Health Board being required to have their own 'Prevent' strategy.
3. For a brief history of the emergence of frameworks, including board certification in the USA, see (Cadge 2012, Chapter 1). In the UK, the healthcare chaplaincy professional associations launched the UK Board for Healthcare Chaplaincy in 2008; see www.ukbhc.org.uk.
4. For a discussion of the theory and practice of chaplaincy offering capital in public negotiation of its role in security and the provision of equal opportunity, in prisons and the Armed Forces, see Todd (2014).
5. Thus the multi-faith space in the new Queen Elizabeth Hospital, Birmingham, which attracted significant public money, is named the 'Faith and Community Centre'.
6. As is apparent from the way a number of spaces are named in relation to this term.
7. For a discussion of some of these issues see Swift (2014, Chapter 4) on 'the Battle of Worcester'.
8. For a discussion of professionalisation of healthcare chaplaincy in the USA, see Cadge (2012), Chapter 5.
9. For an overview and downloadable key publications, see NHS Education Scotland (n.d.).
10. The final report of The Mid Staffordshire NHS Foundation Trust Public Inquiry (2013), chaired by Robert Francis QC.
11. For notes of meeting see AHPCC (2013).
12. Developed as mindfulness-based stress reduction by Jon Kabat-Zinn, or as cognitive mindfulness-based therapy by Mark Williams and others.

CHAPTER 6

Legal and Policy Frameworks for Spiritual Care

Layla Welford

Introduction

The interaction of state law, social policy and religious law in the governance of freedom of religion has long been controversial. The debate surrounding these issues is particularly relevant in state institutions such as hospitals, prisons, schools and the armed forces, where the manifestation of religious beliefs may require the use of limited and valuable state resources, for example, in the provision of religious texts, prayer mats and special foods supplied to meet the needs of religious diets.

This chapter will seek to explore the legal and social policy frameworks in England, Wales and Scotland that govern state-funded chaplaincy within the NHS, with comparative references to systems operative in other institutions and other jurisdictions. Recent research that was conducted at Cardiff University, funded jointly by the Arts and Humanities Research Council and the Economic and Social Research Council, will also be drawn upon before concluding on the suitability of the current frameworks.

In order to fully understand what is prescribed by law, it is necessary to understand how the words used are defined. In this instance, defining what is meant by *religious* and *spiritual* care is helpful. In 2003 the Department of Health issued guidelines for the framework of state-funded chaplaincy within NHS Trusts, and this was followed by similar guidelines being issued in Scotland in 2007 and in Wales in 2010 (hereafter referred to as the Scottish and Welsh guidelines, respectively).

All three documents accept the same definitions of religious and spiritual care, and so for the purposes of this work, the definitions contained within those documents will be adopted,[1] and will be discussed later in the chapter. The 2003 guidelines were renegotiated in 2014 and new guidelines published in 2015 (NHS England 2015). This chapter notes significant continuities and changes, while recognising that the document is not yet in effect. The puzzle, noted in public consultation on the draft, is why the new document should still be 'guidelines', given the statutory framework in effect in Scotland and Wales. The 2015 NHS England guidelines are also discussed in Chapter 5.

The legal framework of religious and spiritual care in hospitals
European law

> *9(1): Everyone has the right to freedom of thought, conscience and religion; this right includes freedom to change his religion or belief and freedom, either alone or in community with others and in public or private, to manifest his religion or belief, in worship, teaching, practice and observance.*
>
> *9(2): Freedom to manifest one's religion or beliefs shall be subject only to such limitations as are prescribed by law and are necessary in a democratic society in the interests of public safety, for the protection of public order, health or morals, or for the protection of the rights and freedoms of others. (Article 9 of the European Convention on Human Rights)*

Article 9 of the European Convention on Human Rights (hereafter referred to as 'ECHR') provides for the right to 'freedom of thought, conscience and religion', and this is an absolute right: there are no qualifications or limitations on the free exercise of this right. The latter part of Article 9(1) provides for freedom to manifest a religion or belief in 'worship, teaching, practice and observance', and such protection is limited to these areas. The right to manifest one's religion or belief is a qualified one, and is subject to the limitations laid down in Article 9(2). These limitations have been tested in case law such as in *X v UK* (1983), where a prisoner was denied attendance at Sunday worship due to the risk of causing disorder at the event.

The European Commission, along with the European Court of Human Rights, seem to have adopted the approach that people should be free to practise their religion, so long as in doing so they do not interfere with the rights and enjoyment of others. Christos Rozakis, one of the vice-presidents of the European Court of Human Rights, stated that 'when balancing the interests of the individual believer' who seeks to 'have their right enforced against the modern, largely secular, democratic society', the interest of the latter lies higher than the interests of the individual applicant (Rozakis 1998). From this, it would appear that the limitations in Article 9(2) are stronger than the rights in Article 9(1).

In France, the doctrine of *laicité positive* requires that there is a 'wall of separation' between religion and the State. However, the State nonetheless considers it a *duty* to provide for the manifestation of religion in places where people are unable to leave (Basdevant-Gaudemet 2005, p.180). This duty exists in order to ensure that the right to freedom of religion is observed. In the UK, therefore, it may be argued that patients who are unable to leave a hospital are entitled to certain measures that ensure their religious freedom, and that there is therefore an implied right under Article 9 of the ECHR to religious care in state hospitals.

Domestic law

Much debate exists over the legal basis of the right to spiritual and religious care in hospitals within domestic law (Doe 2002; Naismith 2001); as such a right is not enshrined clearly in any one single piece of legislation.

It may be argued that the 1998 Human Rights Act gives a legal basis to the right to spiritual care in hospitals, as it incorporates Article 9(1) of the ECHR into domestic law. If individuals are unable to manifest their beliefs whilst in hospital, it is possible that a legal claim could follow. However, to date there has been no litigation on the matter and so it is currently unclear what would happen in the case of a dispute. Furthermore, whilst the right to 'freedom of thought, conscience and religion' is an absolute one, it must be remembered that the right to manifest that right is qualified and subject to the restraints in Article 9(2). A clear example of where limitations are imposed on the exercise of the right under Article 9 of the ECHR is given by Dan Morris, who states that 'a religious terrorist cannot justify his or her actions by appealing to Art.9' (Morris 2003, p.74).

In contrast to the position in hospitals, s.7(1) and s.7(4) of the 1952 Prison Act require all prisons to have at least one Anglican chaplain, and 'an assistant chaplain' where the size of the prison population is large enough to warrant it in the opinion of the Secretary of State. These provisions apply both to State prisons and contracted out prisons,[2] therefore requiring all prisons in England and Wales to have a chaplain.

The early prison system enshrined the idea of chaplains owing a duty to prisoners. Scot Peterson notes that prisons in the USA originated as 'religious institutions', based on the idea that 'inmates could reform if they [...] engage in reflection, prayer, Bible-reading and work, thus establishing a new personal foundation for functioning as productive members of [...] society' (Peterson 2005, p.67). Similarly, s.4 of the Prison Ministers Act 1863 provided that religious books could be distributed throughout prisons in England and Scotland 'as [the chaplain] may deem proper for the religious and moral instruction of prisoners'.

The idea of 'religious medicine' being used in prisons to reform inmates may not be so welcome in today's religiously pluralist society. However, if the World Health Organization's (WHO) definition of health as 'a state of complete physical, mental and social well-being and not merely the absence of disease or infirmity' (WHO 1946) is accepted, then there is no reason why the prison system itself could not be seen as a form of medicine, using rehabilitation as a form of therapy. It is aiming to restore a convicted person to 'health' and to prevent them from re-offending, much like the ideal expressed by Peterson of providing prisoners with a basis that enables them to '[function] as productive members of [...] society' (Peterson 2005, p.67). Similarly, if the NHS is pursing the increase of public health, then it too should be providing for spiritual care if the WHO definition of health is accepted.

While the right to religious care in prisons is enshrined clearly in primary legislation, in hospitals the position is governed through frameworks set out in social policy, to which we now turn.

Social policy frameworks

The Department of Health publication that replaced that Patients' Charter in 2001 provides that the NHS must 'respect [the patient's] religious, spiritual and cultural needs' (Department of Health 2001, s.5). Although this is not a legal right, failure to meet this right 'generally falls within the investigative powers of the health service ombudsman' (Doe 2003, p.189). Furthermore, in 2003 the Department of Health published guidelines for the provision of religious and spiritual care

(Department of Health 2003). These guidelines cover a vast array of aspects of chaplaincy care, from the provision of space for worship to emergency incident planning and bereavement services. However, it must be noted that these are only guidelines, do not constitute legislation, and are therefore unenforceable by law (Welford 2011). Chaplains themselves would, however, be subject to discipline if they breached the 2003 guidelines. It may be noted, however, that chaplains would still be subject to discipline if they breached the 2003 guidelines under the *Health Care Chaplaincy: Code of Conduct* (Association of Hospice and Palliative Care Chaplains 2005).[3]

As has previously been noted, the Department of Health 2003 guidelines were followed by standards being issued in Scotland in 2007 and in Wales in 2010 (NHS Scotland 2007; Welsh Assembly Government 2010). The key distinction that is made in all three sets of guidelines is that between religious care and spiritual care. Spiritual care is seen as something that people of all faith groups and those of no faith can benefit from and have needs for, whereas religious care is restricted to requirements for living in accordance with rules or practices of a recognised religion. The 2003 guidelines provide that, 'references to religion and/or faith are taken to include the nine major world faiths', which are listed as: Bahá'i, Buddhism, Christianity, Hinduism, Jainism, Judaism, Islam, Sikhism and Zoroastrianism (p.5). The guidelines further state that:

> *Spiritual needs may not always be expressed within a religious framework. It is important to be aware that all human beings are spiritual beings who have spiritual needs at different times of their lives. Although spiritual care is not necessarily religious care, religious care, at its best, should always be spiritual. (2003, p.5)[4]*

Similarly, both the Scottish and Welsh guidelines define religious needs as those that arise 'in the context of the shared beliefs, values, liturgies and lifestyle of a faith community' (Standard 1).

As the NHS has explicitly stated that its religious care is only to apply to the nine major world faiths, it is possible in the exercise of Convention rights that a claim could be brought under Article 14 of the ECHR that prohibits discrimination. This would be likely to succeed, for example, where Christian denominations were being afforded privileges that other faiths were not, as for a discrimination claim to succeed it must be shown that there is a comparable group which is being treated more favourably, without justification (*Lithgow v UK* 1986).

However, Article 14 must be invoked alongside another Convention Article in order for a claim to succeed as it does not exist as a right in itself.[5] It cannot be invoked on its own.

Undoubtedly there were issues of both practicalities and funding in mind when the NHS limited its chaplaincy-spiritual care to only include religious care for the nine major world religions, but nonetheless this restriction is inherently discriminatory. The regulatory regime is frozen in time as, although it has been enacted at a time when its provisions were thought to be acceptable, it will remain the same throughout changes in social thinking, and require regular reviews in order to keep in line with public views. Indeed, increasing religious pluralism in the UK influenced the 2015 NHS Chaplaincy Guidelines for NHS England (NHS England 2015), in which the restriction of the number of world faiths is not included. Further, inclusion of increasing diversity of religion and belief is a positive principle in the guidelines:

> The changing nature of communities in England means that chaplains respond to calls of increasing complexity. The diversity of religions and cultures within the population has grown and the need for chaplaincy departments to advise providers about equality and access has increased... In order to put patients first the NHS in England seeks to understand the rich variety of beliefs and values of the population in its care. Chaplains are an essential resource for achieving the ambition to provide high quality care for all and promote the protected characteristics of both religion and belief. (NHS England 2015, p.7)

Calls were also made from the British Humanist Association in 2004 and the National Secular Society in 2010, both of which claim to have equivalent needs to those of religious people that are not being met. It is submitted, however, that such calls have arisen from a lack of understanding of the spiritual care that chaplains provide to all patients and staff, not merely to the religious.

The 2003 guidelines issued by the Department of Health were the first major piece of social policy designed to ensure the equality of chaplaincy services being offered across NHS Trusts. In contrast to this, the 2007 Scottish guidelines and 2010 Welsh guidelines had the benefit of being able to evaluate the efficacy of the existing guidelines, and were therefore able to account for some of the issues that the previous guidance had overlooked, such as the self-assessment tools appended to both of these guidelines, designed for use in auditing chaplaincy services. The Welsh and Scottish guidelines are almost identical except for some minor wording changes, but differ substantially to the 2003 Department of Health guidelines. The Welsh and Scottish guidelines will therefore be referred to together except in specified places where differences arise.

Appointments to chaplaincy posts

The 2003 Department of Health guidelines provide that, 'chaplaincy provision is [to be] made available across the organisation out of normal hours and staffing levels take account of this', and that arrangements are put in place to cater for the 'spiritual, religious sacramental, ritual and cultural requirements appropriate to the needs, background and tradition of all patients and staff, including those of no specified faith'. Appointments to chaplaincy posts are to be made following standard human resource procedures, in partnership with a faith community representative who can 'ensure that the candidates hold the authority of the faith community and can be empowered to act as its representative within the healthcare setting'. Finally, 'appropriate and timely access to services from smaller faith communities is [to be] provided (as well as minorities within faith groups)'. The standard is therefore all-encompassing and far reaching, requiring chaplaincy services across the entire organisation, out of normal hours, for those of all faiths and those of none, as well as for the requirements of various denominations within faith groups. In contrast to this, the Welsh and Scottish guidelines do not focus on appointments to chaplaincy posts, but instead focus on the training and development of chaplains. The 2003 guidelines say little more on this matter than that there should be 'appropriate training and development…available to all members of the chaplaincy-spiritual care team' (2003, p.19).

The 2015 NHS England guidelines reiterate the principle in effect in England of 3.75 hours of chaplaincy care per week for every 35 patients 'matched by religion/belief' (NHS England 2015, p.14). The significant proposal is that this figure should be applied to patients 'not identified with a particular faith or belief system' (NHS England 2015, p.16). Appended to the draft guidelines is a 2011 letter to NHS Trust CEOs regarding the then newly established Panel of Healthcare Chaplaincy Appointment Advisors. This continues the principle of advisors, 'drawn from different religions and faiths' (NHS England 2015, appendix A, p.28).

Standard 6 of both the Welsh and Scottish guidelines deals with the training and development of chaplains, stating that all chaplains should have 'received an induction to their new post (new chaplains appointed 2007 on), undertaken introductory training', and that they should have 'regular appraisals (at least annually) to review professional development and training needs'. The Welsh and Scottish guidelines also provide that chaplaincy services should include 'sufficient hours to meet the spiritual and religious needs of patients, carers, staff and volunteers, including out of hours cover'. The Welsh and Scottish guidelines do not state that a faith representative is required to confirm the standing of a chaplain within the relevant faith community prior to appointment, but do state that a chaplain should be a member of a 'professional chaplaincy association with a code of conduct' such as the Association of Hospice and Palliative Care Chaplains, the College of Health Care Chaplains or the Scottish Association of Chaplains in Healthcare. The 2015 NHS England guidelines have a section on 'Training, Development and Research' (NHS England 2015 pp.25-26), that incorporates some of the Scottish and Welsh framework.

Confidentiality and data protection

At present, very little research has been conducted into the effect of data protection laws on the delivery of chaplaincy care, and as such there is a great lack of literature available for consultation. As will be seen, huge difficulties have been faced by healthcare chaplains due to confusion surrounding data protection laws.

The Data Protection Act 1998 (hereafter referred to as the DPA) sets out to regulate the processing of personal data, and lists eight principles that must be adhered to in order for the processing of personal data to be undertaken lawfully. A person's religious affiliation falls within the category of 'sensitive personal data' within the Act, and is therefore subject to more stringent criteria for processing, and is subject to the requirements laid down in Schedule 3 of the Act. This includes the provision that sensitive personal data can be processed for 'medical purposes', and defines 'medical purposes' as including 'preventative medicine, medical diagnosis, medical research, the provision of care and treatment and the management of healthcare services' (schedule 3(2)).

In light of the DPA, concerns arose as to whether members of staff could lawfully pass on details of a patient's religious affiliation to the chaplaincy-spiritual care team, due to the classification of religious affiliation as 'sensitive personal data'. This question was passed for consideration to the Information Commissioner, who concluded that the work of chaplains was not included within the definition of 'medical purposes' under the Schedule 3 exemptions. Furthermore, the definition of 'health professional' in the DPA does not include healthcare chaplains within s.69. This stands in contrast to an increasingly prevalent view amongst healthcare chaplains today that they are both faith practitioners and healthcare professionals, being increasingly subject to NHS requirements in relation to their conduct, accountability, training, pay and benefits, career development, and so on.

The confusion surrounding the DPA laws was only confounded by the Information Commissioner's decision, which is in dire need of review. All three sets of national guidelines clearly state that healthcare chaplains are a vital and integral part of the healthcare team.

Two key problems have resulted from the confusion surrounding the DPA laws. One is the failure to pass on a patient's religious affiliation to the chaplaincy team through fear of breaching the law, and the other is a refusal in some instances to allow chaplains to have access to patient records. The approaches taken vary from Trust to Trust with little coherence in accepted practice. The effect of this not only places chaplains at potential risk, but could also result in chaplains taking steps that undermine therapeutic care, for example, in mental health care services, because they are simply unaware of the patient's needs. A startling example of where chaplains were placed at risk was found in doctoral research in 2011, which reported a case where a patient with AIDS was spitting at people (Welford 2011, p.195). The only way in which the chaplain was aware of the patients' condition was as a result of overhearing a staff conversation a few days previously. The chaplain had been denied access to patient records and was therefore placed at an unnecessary and unacceptable risk. It would appear that consideration in these Trusts has only been given to one side of the coin, i.e. to the consequences of breaching DPA laws. What has not been given sufficient weight is consideration of the risks in which chaplains are being placed in such circumstances.

In an attempt to address this issue, both the Welsh and the Scottish guidelines state that chaplaincy services should have 'access to patient information systems for providing and facilitating appropriate spiritual or religious care and recording information and interventions'. Whilst such a standpoint may be open to challenge given the Information Commissioners' ruling, it nonetheless ensures that chaplains are better placed to be enabled to provide appropriate care within safe boundaries. It also ensures consistency across Trusts, something that the NHS in England currently lacks in this area.

The 2003 Department of Health guidelines state that Trusts '*may* inform patients about the availability of chaplaincy services, for example through information leaflets and "welcome packs"' (p.12, emphasis added). In contrast to this suggestion, the Welsh and Scottish guidelines both state a requirement that 'all patients receive written information on admission containing details of the chaplaincy service available within the unit', with the Welsh guidelines also making provision for such information to be provided 'in an appropriate language'. Given the confusion and fear surrounding the passing on of patient information to chaplaincy teams, such a standard is essential in ensuring that patients are made aware of the chaplaincy services available. The 2003 guidelines reported that Nottingham University Hospital NHS Trust found that the effort to provide such literature 'paid dividends in terms of there being a raising of [the] service's general profile', and, 'helped to more readily identify the service as a general resource for both patients and staff' (p.13).

The extent to which this affects the work of healthcare chaplains was demonstrated in recent research that reported that a Roman Catholic healthcare chaplain was virtually unable to work due to a ruling from the diocesan Bishop that the Roman Catholic chaplains were only to visit Roman Catholic patients, but without being allowed access to patient records it became near impossible for the chaplains to carry out any work because of the combined effect of state law and religious law (Welford 2011)

The 2015 NHS England guidelines create the opportunity for a number of these issues to be resolved, but do not themselves resolve them:

> *All NHS staff requires access to the information needed to carry out their duties. Access to appropriate information is essential for chaplains to provide excellent spiritual care. Such access is subject to strict legal rules and NHS policies which must be observed by all staff. (NHS England 2015, p.24)*

Worship spaces and religious dietary requirements

The 2003 guidelines provide that all NHS Trusts should provide 'accessible and suitable spaces for prayer, reflection and religious services which are open to patients and staff 24 hours a day'. They further state that more than one space may be necessary, and that care needs to be taken when considering furnishings and religious symbolism in order to ensure that the space is suitable for use by different faith groups. The Welsh and Scottish guidelines simply state that there should be 'access to a chapel or prayer room acceptable for the religious observance of all faiths'. The 2015 NHS England guidelines include provision for spaces for 'worship; prayer; contemplation; reflection; stillness and peace' under the heading 'Multi-Faith and Belief Rooms', as a requirement 'in order for human rights and equality to be observed' (NHS England 2015, p.27) The 2003 guidelines also somewhat strangely include the provision of a religious diet under this heading. Conversely, the Welsh and Scottish guidelines fail to deal with this altogether, save under Standard 3 where it is recommended that each Trust have a manual outlining the beliefs and practices of the 'major faith communities and belief groups', which amongst a raft of other things should include 'religious/belief needs that have implications for the patient's stay and well being, e.g. diet, prayer rites and ceremonies'.[6]

There is a vacuum of literature available for consultation with regard to the provision of religious dietary requirements in NHS hospitals in England, Scotland and Wales. However, one particular model is worthy of note by way of comparison. In the USA, the prison service provides a diet called the 'Common Fare' diet. Any prisoner who wishes to avoid certain foods due to religious conviction can go on the diet. The diet itself is fairly basic, but it is suitable for virtually all religious needs (Beckford and Gilliat 1998, p.188). It provides meat dishes three times per week, and the meat itself is kosher. This not only caters for Jews, but also for Muslims, as although the meat is not strictly *Halal*, it is slaughtered by 'people from the Book' (Jews and Christians) and is therefore acceptable to most Muslims. For those who wish to completely abstain from meat, when the meat dishes are provided they can choose to take food from the salad bar instead. Such a model would be relatively straightforward to implement within hospitals, and would remove differences that may exist in the provision between different Trusts due to demographic differences – the only change would need to be the quantity supplied.

Bereavement services and major incident planning

The 2003 Department of Health guidelines recognise that 'chaplaincy-spiritual care is central to providing support and assistance to the bereaved. All NHS Trusts should ensure that the dying and recently bereaved are able to access chaplaincy services.' The Welsh and Scottish guidelines state that chaplaincy services have a 'significant contribution' to make in offering 'spiritual and religious support to the injured or dying', but this is placed within the context of major incidents (Standard 7).

The effect of the law on the work of healthcare chaplains

Recent research at Cardiff University, which was funded jointly by the Arts and Humanities Research Council and the Economic and Social Research Council under their joint Religion and Society funding programme (www.religionandsociety.org.uk), sought to consider the impact that the law has on the work of chaplains on the ground. The work began with an exploration of the existing legal and social policy frameworks before moving on to empirical research that was conducted to examine the efficacy of the existing guidelines, and to what extent the guidelines were being adhered to in practice throughout different Trusts.

Religious dietary requirements

Although religious dietary requirements do not feature within the 2003 Department of Health guidelines, the aforementioned empirical research showed that on the whole, Trusts do cater for religious dietary needs, with 91 per cent of questionnaire respondents affirming that religious dietary requirements are met by their particular Trust. In response to the question of whether there have been any difficulties in meeting these needs, 17.6 per cent indicated that there had been problems, 36.8 per cent that there had not and the remaining 45.6 per cent were not sure. Further research in this area is necessary in order to ascertain whether improvement is needed. What can be suggested, however, is that guidance should be drawn up and circulated around Trusts informing them of the needs of each of the nine major world religions that the 2003 Guidelines state Trusts should cater for. This could be done in the same manner as it has been in prisons, and could help educate and enable better provision to be given. It is likely that providing different diets for each of the nine major world faiths may be costly, and the Common Fare Diet that exists in the USA in prisons may be a model worth aspiring to.

Data protection and confidentiality

The current situation regarding healthcare chaplaincy and data protection is not acceptable. Clear guidance must be issued as a matter of urgency setting out in clear terms what may and may not lawfully be passed on to the chaplaincy team. Information such as a patients' location within a hospital, whether or not they have been discharged, and so on, is not barred under the law, yet the aforementioned research from Cardiff University found that due to confusion and fear of getting it wrong staff are often refusing chaplains this kind of information (Welford, 2011).

It is imperative that the Information Commissioners' decision is challenged, as consideration must be given to the risks that are inadvertently being created by denying chaplains access to key information. Reports of chaplains being put at risk because of a refusal to give information are worrying. The NHS employs chaplains as part of the healthcare team, yet following this ruling they are treated separately to the rest of the team. It seems only common sense that this should be reviewed as it is causing frustration for chaplains, and confusion for patients, their families and other members of staff.

The legal status of the 2003 guidelines

The empirical research discovered that many respondents felt that they would be in a far better position if there were a legal obligation for NHS Trusts to provide chaplaincy services. On the one hand, a legal requirement would at least go some way in ensuring that chaplaincy is provided in the same manner nationwide, and the disparity that currently exists between Trusts would to a large extent be eliminated. However, once this is enshrined in law it in many ways becomes rigid and inflexible, and, given the fast rate at which the religious beliefs of the population are changing, it may in fact be beneficial to continue without a legal requirement for the time being. This is illustrated well by reference to the 1952 Prison Act provisions that deal with prison chaplaincy. The 1952 Act created a legal obligation for all prisons to have at least one Anglican chaplaincy. However, over the past 50 years there has been tremendous growth in religious pluralism, and requiring chaplaincy by law only for the Christian faith is an outdated provision.

The danger, however, in failing to create a legal requirement is that chaplaincy often seems to be an area that comes under scrutiny when budget cuts have to be made. It is essential that the importance of chaplaincy care as part of the holistic care that the NHS provides is not seen as dispensable.

A common complaint by the respondents in the empirical research was that they felt that their Trust did not take them seriously, or did not consider their needs to be important. It could be argued that there would be greater potential for changing such views if a legal requirement were to be created, as Trusts would be in a position of potential liability if they failed to meet that obligation.

Conclusion

Both social policy and the law have a tremendous ability to control the day-to-day work of healthcare chaplains. They can be used to enrich and protect the work of chaplains, but without proper consideration can also create huge barriers to the work.

Chaplains would do well to engage in further empirical research and study that seeks to demonstrate the efficacy of healthcare chaplaincy. Nationwide training or information leaflets would also be beneficial for informing chaplains and other members of the healthcare team of the law, so that chaplains can work without unnecessary hindrances created by a lack of awareness from draftsmen, and other healthcare staff can handle patient information with confidence.

Up until now, it seems that conversations between healthcare chaplains and policy makers have remained minimal, with chaplains failing to recognise the effect that the legal and social policy frameworks are having on them day to day, and policy makers not always seeing the practical effects of their decisions. What is needed is greater communication between these two parties. Social policy can be a useful tool for chaplains when it is written in a way that supports their work, but without proper care and consideration, as with the law, can be a difficult creature to overcome.

Notes

1. However, numerous texts have been devoted to the meaning of such words; see e.g. Carr (2001), Durkheim (1912/2001), Elkins *et al.* (1988) and Mowat and Swinton (2005).

2. The Criminal Justice Act 1991, s.84, states that contracted out prisons are to be run, 'subject to and in accordance with sections 85 and 6 below, the 1952 Act (as modified by section 87 below) and prison rules'. Sections 85 and 86 of the said Act create minor amendments to the 1952 Act such as changes to terminology, i.e. 'prisoner' in the 1952 Act is to be interpreted as 'remand prisoner' when applied to contracted out prisons. Section 86 of the 1991 Act also modifies the powers which officers in contracted out prisons hold. Aside from these modifications, the 1952 Act applies in full force to contracted out prisons, therefore meaning that all state and contracted out prisons are required to have a chaplain in accordance with the requirements stipulated in the 1952 Act.

3. This code has been to some extent succeeded by the UK Board of Healthcare Chaplaincy Code of Conduct published in 2010 and revised in 2012 and 2014.

4. Similar understandings are to be found in the draft 2014 NHS Chaplaincy Guidelines for NHS England: '*Spiritual care* is care provided in the context of illness which addresses the expressed spiritual needs of patients, staff and service users. These needs are likely to include one or more of the following: existential concerns; religious convictions and practices; relationships of significance; and the exploration of faith or belief' (NHS England 2014, introductory definition).

5. Article 14 of the ECHR prohibits discrimination in relation to the enjoyment of the Convention's rights and freedoms, and therefore only applies to discrimination falling within one of the other Convention Articles. It cannot be invoked on its own, and must be invoked alongside another Convention right. However, there need not be a substantive violation of another Article for it to succeed (*Belgian Linguistics Case No 2* 1979 1 EHRR 252), it is enough that it falls within the ambit of a Convention right. See Ovey and White (2006), p.415 for a more detailed discussion.

6. The draft NHS England guidelines make no mention of diet in relation to religious belief.

CHAPTER 7

From Atheists to Zoroastrians...

What are the Implications for Professional Healthcare Chaplaincy of the Requirement to Provide Spiritual Care to People of All Faiths and None?

Mirabai Galashan

Introduction

Webster's Dictionary defines 'chaplain' as:

1. A clergyman in charge of a chapel.

2. A clergyman officially attached to a branch of the military, to an institution, or to a family or court.

3. A person chosen to conduct religious exercises (as at a meeting of a club or society).

4. A clergyman appointed to assist a bishop (as at a liturgical function) (emphasis added).

(Rights 2009, article on 'chaplain')

The role and person of the postmodern healthcare chaplain has changed almost beyond recognition from these definitions. Once a religious figure assigned to minister to the faithful of her community, the postmodern healthcare chaplain is a professional employed by or through a secular institution to fulfil a mandate to provide the spiritual care to which all patients are equally entitled. This situation in which chaplaincy currently finds itself may be attributed in large part to the convergence of a number of social, religious, cultural and political issues. One starting point is offered by McCarthy, who describes the post-modern consciousness as an increasing focus on the relativity and particularity of every perspective and position (2000, p.198). This phenomenon can be observed with particular clarity in relation to the sphere of religious and spiritual identity in contemporary culture. Thus, while many people equate spirituality with religion, the terms are no longer synonymous, though still conceptually related (Sulmasy 2006, p.13). If spirituality were allowed to be defined only synonymously with religion and a belief in God, then several groups of persons – namely atheists, agnostics, humanists and hedonists – would be excluded from using spiritual coping mechanisms. Therefore, spirituality should apply to both believers and non-believers (Anderson 2004; Baldacchino and Draper 2001) and since the purpose of a healthcare chaplain is to provide spiritual care to *all* patients, by definition this work cannot be restricted to serving those who subscribe to a particular, or indeed to *any*, religious faith. Hence we have the unique paradox of the contemporary chaplain: a person identified by her faithful adherence to one particular religious tradition, tasked with ministering to the spiritual needs of a multitude comprising those of all faiths and those with no (and no traditional) faith. This chapter explores the implications of the changed context in which healthcare chaplaincy finds itself. It further argues that important and challenging work is still to be done if chaplaincy is to offer a fully inclusive practice.

Changing patterns of religion and spirituality

Central to the argument of the chapter, as indicated previously, is the cultural hybridity of the context in which chaplains seek to practise. The impact of globalisation has led to a dissolution of boundaries, allowing the free traffic of ideas, media, people and capital, and resulting in an increasingly heterogeneous religious terrain (Vasquez and Marquardt 2003). The 2008 *US Religious Landscape Survey* revealed that whilst America was still a predominantly Christian society (78%), religious affiliation in the US was both very diverse and extremely fluid (Pew Forum on Religion and Public Life 2008, p.5).

One of the most significant developments has been the emergence and burgeoning of the 'Nones', people who describe themselves as affiliated with no particular faith. According to Gallup in 1950 only 2 per cent of the population described themselves as unaffiliated with any religion; in 2012, that number reached 17.8 per cent (Gallup Daily Tracking 2012). The Pew Forum on Religion and Public Life put the figure even higher at 19.6 per cent and revealed that one-third of young people under 30 are 'Nones' (Pew Forum on Religion and Public Life 2012).

However, these facts should not be misconstrued to mean that the US is becoming a secular nation. Of those unaffiliated with a particular religion, two-thirds say they believe in God (68%). More than half say they often feel a deep connection with nature and the earth (58%), while more than a third classify themselves as 'spiritual' but not 'religious' (37%), and one in five (21%) say they 'pray every day' (Pew Forum on Religion and Public Life 2012). What this strongly suggests is a rejection of the organisational and social structures that form the architecture of traditional organisations (including religious ones).

In spite of its characterisation as one of the most secular countries in the world (Brierly cited in Paley 2008), there is a similar trend in the UK (Coleman, Ivani-Chalian and Robinson 2004). Whilst some people may not be overtly religious or attend worship services, nonetheless they still participate in an existential and spiritual search for meaning (Speck 2004). Davie (1990) identified this trend as 'believing without belonging' and Swift (2009, p.1) calls it the 'effective de-regulating of spiritual experience amongst the population at large'. Underwood and Teresi (2002) simply refer to this significant sector of the population as 'spiritual but not religious'.

Religion and spirituality in healthcare

The above phenomenon is reflected amongst physicians in the USA. In a study, while 64 per cent of doctors said that they thought of themselves as *spiritual*, only 30 per cent actually engaged in organised religion either regularly or occasionally, and 34 per cent described themselves as being spiritual but not involved with any religious group (Curlin *et al.* 2005).

This newfound significance of spirituality in healthcare reflects the de-traditionalisation and the individualisation of religion expressed in a 'culture of choice' in which people now feel they may choose and create their own 'religions' (Woodhead and Heelas 2000, p.345).

A 2002 analysis of healthcare literature found 92 definitions of *spirituality* and identified seven subcategories of meaning:

1. relationship to God, spiritual being, higher power, a reality greater than the self

2. not of the self

3. transcendence or connectedness unrelated to a belief in a higher being

4. existential, not of the material world

5. meaning and purpose in life

6. life force of the person, integrating aspect of the person

7. summative (combining multiple features of spirituality).

(Unruh, Versnel and Kerr 2002)

It is significant that only one of these seven sub-categories refers to God or a higher being. Spirituality in healthcare is increasingly being defined in apophatic terms in relationship to religion. Berlinger succinctly exemplifies this challenge in her apology to Foucault: '[A]pologies to Foucault... I who conduct this discourse am *not* conducting a religious discourse, I am *not* promoting religion' (emphasis in the original) (2004, p. 683).

A national survey of hospital chaplains undertaken in Sweden identified that only 8 per cent of questions posed to chaplains centred on religious issues (Strang and Strang 2002). Two studies by McGrath found that staying intimately connected with life through family, home, friends, leisure and work is just as vital spiritually to individuals as is transcendent meaning-making (McGrath 2003a, 2003b). Another study demonstrated the potential for using a modified spirituality model to assess, intervene and evaluate interventions for atheists (Smith-Stoner 2007).

The development toward decentralised spirituality, along with the idea that people who are both humanists and atheists have begun to articulate a belief in 'the spiritual' (Holloway 2006, p.836), is a critical issue in the discourse regarding the future of healthcare chaplaincy.

Implications for healthcare chaplaincy

This pursuit of a definition for spirituality, and the ensuing adoption of the concept as a universal *need* or *right* in healthcare, raises the question of who should meet that need. Academic literature confirms that it is not just chaplains, but also physicians, nurses, social workers and others, who are examining their roles in relation to spirituality and spiritual care. For example, the Royal College of Psychiatrists defines spirituality in the healthcare context as being identified with experiencing a deep sense of meaning and purpose in life, accompanied by a sense of belonging, acceptance, integration and wholeness (Lachlan 2008). This widespread interest in spiritual care is a double-edged sword for chaplaincy: the global financial crisis in healthcare has created scarcity-driven competition for funding among allied health professions and there is no clear delineation that the domain and the provision of this care is solely within the provenance of the chaplain.

Chaplains practice in the liminal space between faith and science. The need to justify their continued existence in the world of evidence-based medicine has been a catalyst towards professionalisation. Professional bodies have been formed, with standards of competence and qualifications coalescing both from within the profession and from regulatory bodies. The need to participate in more academically rigorous clinical research has been articulated internationally by chaplaincy organisations, educational institutions and in journals.

The above are aspects of chaplains seeking to redefine themselves as clinical professionals rather than visiting clergy, and to justify their continued existence in the climate of evidence-based medicine. Central to this quest is the question of what makes them uniquely qualified to deliver spiritual care. The clearest evidence for this being a central concern is the emergence of the focus on generating clinical research in healthcare chaplaincy, exhibited in professional curricula, research grants and publications.

Referring to the intense interest in the subject within the related area of nursing literature, Paley suggests the very act of seeking a definition for spirituality in healthcare is not an innocent philosophical or academic pursuit. He refers to it as a 'propaganda exercise (in a non-pejorative sense) rather than an exercise in conceptual analysis' (2008, p.176). Nurses are thus engaged in their own professionalisation project regarding spiritual care, in which they stake 'a claim to jurisdiction over a newly invented sphere of work' (Paley 2008, p.175). This use of the concept of spirituality is elastic; the purpose of the ever-expanding range of definitions of experiences that are considered 'spiritual' is not necessarily to *identify* spiritual needs, but to create them and name them as part of their own remit (Paley 2008, p.179).

Chaplaincy on the threshold

This chapter argues that healthcare chaplaincy resides in a state of jurisdictional liminality, which is derived from the fact that it has detached itself from its origins within the sphere of religious control, but has yet to find secure moorings in secular frameworks of organisation. In the USA, chaplains are now routinely employed to provide spiritual care to an increasingly diverse patient body. The emerging distinction between pastoral care and sacramental function allows the chaplain to meet many of the spiritual needs of those of other faiths and to call upon the services of representative clergy to provide the particular ritual functions required. This separation, furthermore, invites expanded definitions of pastoral care to meet the needs of those with no faith and gives rise to approaches known as *generic care*. The term demonstrates the intention to embrace diversity. But it is not value-free and the approaches are contested. Indeed it is precisely in this context that a number of issues arise centred on the competing forces that seek to control and dominate the practice of chaplaincy.

Chaplaincy qualifications

One of the corollaries of generic spiritual care for all is the need to challenge the relevance of qualifications and training for the profession. This is particularly the case where qualifications are anachronistically still defined by specifically, and almost exclusively religious requirements, reflecting the historical precedent of the role rather than the modern practice of the healthcare chaplain.

Current uncertainty is reflected in the absence of unified qualifications and standardised training, independent of the theological training that is often a prerequisite for obtaining a job in healthcare chaplaincy. Various agencies create and promote their own competing standards, certifications and subsidiary agencies. The USA does utilise a widespread system of specialised training, clinical pastoral education (CPE), designed to equip chaplains to deal with crisis situations, respond to all persons with equal sensitivity and compassion, and to function within a multidisciplinary team network in an institutional setting (Snorton 2006). CPE benefits from an action–reflection learning approach similar to other graduate medical education, giving students the opportunity to work with patients whilst they are training.

Two key arguments for such training are to: (i) prepare chaplains for ministry in culturally diverse settings; and (ii) to protect clients from those who are well intentioned, but who remain untrained. The perceived danger of being untrained is that they might proselytise amongst the patients when their job is instead to listen respectfully to the spiritual: the worries, the fears, the anger and the overall emotions and experiences of the patients they serve (Snorton 2006, pp.661–662). Craddock Lee (2002) concurs that secularised, professional training in the form of CPE enables the transformation of chaplaincy from a peripheral service that is truly only beneficial to a small minority of religious patients, into an integral element of universal patient care.

But such training only partly answers the question, arising from the prevalence of non-religious meanings of spiritual care, of whether the current selection, training and methodologies utilised by healthcare chaplaincy are appropriate for the delivery of a largely non-religious practice. Chaplaincy still uses the religious qualification as a means to name and own the expertise of spiritual care and justify their position as the rightful providers of such care in the face of the challenge that spiritual care in healthcare may be equally the role, duty or capability of other professions, namely nurses, social workers or psychologists; and in the face of the view that this religio-centric paradigm could in fact be disadvantageous.

> *Indeed it is precisely because of their specifically religious origins and training that chaplains as representatives of particular religious views and communities may be the last people suitable for facilitating or providing 'spiritual care' in the generic secularised sense that seems now to be prevalent across a variety of professions (Pattison 2001, p.34).*

Lack of diversity within the profession

Yet another issue arising from the requirement to provide spiritual care across a multitude of spiritual and religious identities is the lack of diversity within the profession. At present, there are many spiritual minorities that are severely underrepresented in healthcare chaplaincy, and some, such as Native Americans, atheists, pagans and humanists, may be entirely unrepresented due to credentialing restrictions.

Writing about the increasingly formal inclusion of spirituality in medical school curriculum, Nancy Berlinger asks some pertinent questions that highlight these concerns. Which definitions of spirituality are promoted? Which tenets of spirituality and education are certifiable, and which are simply matters of faith? (2004, p.681).

The 1996 examination of chaplaincy in the NHS and its response to religious diversification by Beckford and Gilliat noted a strong element of paternalism and distinguished between inclusion *by right* and *by concession* (1996, p.508). Systems where work was assigned by proportionality were seen as detrimental to local faith minorities, and faiths that lacked centralised management were at a disadvantage (Swift 2009, p.50).

The challenge for healthcare chaplaincy is to avoid replicating the pervasive cultural stigmatisation of certain faith or no-faith groups by the dominant traditions. One of the major problems of having the future of chaplaincy debated only by the current stakeholders is the risk that the interests of minorities are not being represented. It is to be hoped that the ongoing professionalisation of healthcare chaplaincy will avoid what Lane (2006) refers to as Abbott's identified strategy of usurpation of power through 'cultural work' that:

> [A]ctively maintains separate professional spheres and shores up the boundaries of the dominant group [by] claiming a public service ethos over pecuniary self-interest and labeling competitor groups as amateurs or 'snake oil merchants.' Such strategies stigmatize the 'other' and simultaneously create a sense of anxiety and fear in the public. (Abbott 1988, p.342)

In the USA, the Association of Professional Chaplains has been receptive to a call from grassroots members to consider the interests of groups not currently represented or underrepresented. In 2012, the author led one of two taskforces that were created to look at the educational and endorsement requirements for board certification and to make recommendations and suggestions for how the Association might respond to a growing minority of chaplains who would not currently be eligible for board certification due to a non-traditional education and affiliation.

In the USA, whilst it is still technically possible to get a job as a humanist or atheist chaplain as long as you have at least some units of CPE, board certification is out of reach without endorsement by a 'recognised faith tradition'. Interestingly, there is a distinction in the requirements of hospice, as opposed to hospital employers. Hospital chaplain positions increasingly require board certification or eligibility to become board certified within two or three years, in addition to a graduate theological degree and endorsement. But a 2012 study of US hospice chaplain job advertisements revealed 'that 44% of chaplain job advertisements did not require chaplain applicants to have completed clinical pastoral education (CPE) and 41% did not require ordination and/or endorsement from a recognized denomination. Only 37% of hiring organizations required or preferred professional certification' (Cramer and Tenzek 2012).

Whilst in a demographic sense, the UK is more secular than the USA; its chaplaincy is still more closely aligned with religion. In the UK, the requirement for employment as a healthcare chaplain still normally requires ordination and endorsement by a 'recognised' faith group and quite often there is a specification of denomination as illustrated in this advertisement for a part-time chaplain for the NHS:

> *There is an anticipated commitment to the spiritual care of all regardless of faith or culture. The applicant should be ordained and licensed by Bishop (or equivalent, if Free Church/Non Christian faith, and have a minimum of 2 years' experience of ordained ministry. (NHS job site 2009)*

Historically, chaplaincy was organised along parochial lines and, in the UK, there are more obvious vestiges from the 'proportional representation' school of chaplaincy, which was able to meet spiritual care needs by employing appropriate representatives of the faiths of the patients. The continued attempt to organise pastoral care in this way is not an option for the future, as it would be both entirely cost-prohibitive and wildly impractical for every healthcare institution to have on hand a representative of every religious and/or spiritual identity to which a patient might ascribe. Aside from the logistic impossibility of employing a fraction of a percentage of a Zoroastrian chaplain at each institution, this would also raise the question of who would cater to the spiritual needs of non-religious patients, given the current barriers to the profession faced by atheists and humanists.

Nolan (2008), writing from the UK, feels that the profession is limited by the perception that spiritual care is equal to religious care. He describes the paradox facing the NHS chaplain who is employed on a parochial basis. To secure a chaplaincy post, the chaplain must be endorsed by a particular religious organisation. Swift sees the continued specification of denomination in job advertisements leading to a hampering of the open market (2009, p.77). Eliminating this bias would raise the general quality of applicants and Swift adds there is no evidence that demonstrates chaplains of particular denominations or faiths can better serve patients of another denomination, or that patients are more or less satisfied with care from a minister from any particular denomination (2009, p.77).

Nolan agrees this professional protectionism of healthcare chaplaincy, which champions religious endorsement as a qualification to practise, is inherently dangerous to the profession since, when resources are scarce, it would support the idea that spiritual care can be outsourced (Nolan 2008). This situation describes two opposing agendas that simultaneously exist in conflict within the profession. First, the desire to categorise the work as 'spiritual care' in order to make the chaplain eligible to work with all patients, thus adding value to the organisation and shoring up the justification for the job's existence. But second, the profession wants to insist that the only persons who can join in this work, 'must, like me, be recognized by a faith community' (Nolan 2008). The process of emphasising that the nature of the work is, indeed, *spiritual*, whilst policing the boundaries of the profession by insisting on religious affiliation, merely strengthens 'the misconception that we operate primarily as religious officiants, addressing primarily religious needs' (Nolan 2008).

Nolan (2008) suggests an approach that retains endorsement by a religious authority, yet is careful to explain its relevance. He asserts that it is not being trained in practices that pertain to a particular religious tradition that qualifies one as a chaplain, but the attendant training and experience in spiritual development that 'equips us to be with others who are going through a period of intense spiritual crisis' (Nolan 2008).

One of the most impressive achievements within the framework established by the Scottish Executive Health Department (2002) was the encapsulation of a working philosophy that delineated the scope of chaplaincy in relation to both those with, and those without religious beliefs. This policy statement addresses various non-religious, yet vital, functions of the chaplain:

- as a provider of support in times of crisis

- as a facilitator to assist in addressing the search for meaning

- as an aid to help cope with suffering, loss, fear, loneliness, anxiety, uncertainty, impairment, despair, anger and guilt

- as a counselor in ethical dilemmas

- as a skilled and sensitive listener who has time to be with those who are suffering

- as a witness to deep spiritual stirrings and desires of the patient's spirit and the significance of their personal relationships

- as a validator

- as a person who empowers others to find within themselves the resources to cope with their difficulties and the capacity to make positive use of their experience of illness and injury.

(Scottish Executive Health Department 2002)

These six skills use the term *faith*, while the terms *religion* or *religious* are notably, and appropriately, absent. This list of requirements passes the ultimate litmus test of inclusivity in that an atheist chaplain would actually be able to fulfil these criteria. The transformation of the role and the person of the chaplain, from religious functionary to spiritual care-giver, is illuminated by the emphasis on *relational* rather than *didactic* skills and competencies.

The appreciation of the idea that the profession of chaplaincy requires certain traits of character and behaviour, which are easily excluded from a technical approach to quantifying skill as a byproduct of education, or dependent on religion, is an approach that is to be both commended and recommended. This is an issue that needs to be addressed throughout the profession, as qualifications and training are reexamined in light of the changing job description of the chaplain.

Protecting against risk

Operating in a notoriously litigious society, US healthcare institutions are naturally eager to utilise any means possible to indemnify themselves against the risk of a malpractice suit. Hence, they are happy to delegate some of the responsibility to a professional association. In turn, the healthcare chaplaincy associations employ the mechanism of requiring 'endorsement' by a religious body to relieve themselves of some of the responsibility for screening practitioners.

If the purpose of the requirement of endorsement by a faith tradition is to protect the public from incompetent or malicious practitioners, this practice may be inherently flawed due to its basis on certain assumptions. First, a level of parity is assumed in the standards that endorsers utilise. Second, it is assumed that each of the endorsing traditions operates a screening system with criteria relevant to the competencies and skills most appropriate to chaplaincy, rather than ministry. Arguably, these are not only very different, but may in fact be in direct conflict. Engelhardt notes how poorly:

> [t]raditional Christianity fits within contemporary commitments to inclusiveness and tolerance that characterize contemporary Western Culture… [O]nce chaplaincy is defined by fully ecumenical professional norms, justifiable within the discourse of a secular space, chaplaincy takes on an identity independent of and hostile to traditional Christian concerns. (Engelhardt 2003, p.140)

Given that the most commonly cited example of 'dangerous' practice in chaplaincy is that of proselytisation, it seems somewhat counterintuitive to favour those in receipt of the stamp of approval to serve as an ordained representative of a particular faith tradition. Since, 'the proclamation of the good news of the redemption by the Son of God, the Messiah of Israel, implicitly criticizes the religion and bioethics of others' (Engelhardt 2003, p.140), logically speaking, it would follow that the public would be afforded the greatest protection from spiritual abuse by being served by chaplains tied to no particular faith (i.e. atheists and agnostics).

Viewed through a neo-Weberian lens, the movement towards professionalisation may also be seen as an act of exclusionary occupational closure, designed to establish a monopolistic control of the employment opportunities for chaplains (Woodward in Orchard 2001, p.86). The chief concern lies in the potential for the current ruling class in chaplaincy to use professionalisation as an opportunity to secure and enhance its privileged access to rewards and opportunities in the labour market. By *ruling class*, reference is made to the identity of the groups who currently uphold themselves as speaking for the profession, whose race, gender, religious identification and class are, arguably, far from representative of the demographics of the populations they serve. The effect of this is captured, in relation to a different context, by Sword.

> *Professionalization under the guise of public protection seems to really be protection for the self-interest of the practitioner. It will keep the untrained – by our definition – out of the practice thus excluding the elders, the community workers, the intuitive naturals, those with stature in their cultures and others who have been doing the work for years without recognition or credit for the value of the work they are doing. It will marginalize those who cannot pay the thousands of dollars to be steeped in our standard model that barely recognizes the voices of the other gender, cultures, races, classes, experiences or locations. (Sword 2009)*

Chaplains, as they pursue equal status with other allied health providers, such as social workers, are the only professionals whose certification is not solely based on education or competency, but require the endorsement by sectarians of core religious beliefs (Brassey, 2009).

Chaplaincy endorsement

One of the issues that board certification raises is that qualification is determined not merely on skills and competencies but on endorsement by a faith group or 'a demonstrated connection to a recognized religious community' (Association of Professional Chaplains *et al.* 2001). The list of endorsing bodies reflects the mainstream religious traditions, as previously discussed. This effectively creates significant barriers to minority faith traditions, to those of no faith and to the *spiritual but not religious*, in particular.

In the USA, religious freedom is one of the most fundamental rights protected by the constitution (ACLU 2014). The right to believe (or to not believe), the right to express and to manifest religious beliefs, and the right to be free *from* religion are all guaranteed by the First Amendment's Free Exercise and Establishment clauses (ACLU 2008).

Brassey (2009) is amongst those who campaign for a single certifying body to end these inequalities that exclude gifted, trained and qualified candidates on the grounds that their spiritual path has not led them through a denominational structure, or because their personal journey has led them in a different direction from that of their chosen faith. He condemns a practice that offers chaplains the choice of lying in order to receive endorsement, forced to conceal something that has nothing to do with their skills, competencies, education or experience in providing pastoral care.

The argument is that chaplains desire recognition as full, professional members of our healthcare teams. Yet, they remain the only members of those teams whose certification is based, in part, on something other than education or competency – the endorsement by religious bodies. The dominance of the religious 'ruling class' is reflected in the innate bias espoused by the professional associations that are the current controlling interest in healthcare chaplaincy. There is a moral antithesis between the requirement as a chaplain to serve regardless of cultural, social and spiritual identity, and the requirement to demonstrate eligibility for this role by achieving endorsement from a body that may espouse proselytisation and condemnation of persons with whom they disagree (Brassey 2009). Ironically, therefore, if the 'promotion of generic, religiously neutral spiritual care is the ideal in healthcare, then nurses, existential counselors, or philosophers might be better suited to providing care and assistance than chaplains' (Pattison 2001, p.34).

Defining chaplaincy as *spiritual* rather than *religious* care, challenges the idea that spiritual care is the role of a provider defined and qualified by a specifically religious expertise. The transformation of the role and the person of the healthcare chaplain from religious functionary to spiritual care-giver should be illuminated by the emphasis on *relational* rather than *didactic* skills and competencies. The post-modern healthcare chaplain does not administer prescriptions for physical or spiritual health – her role is not so much to intervene, advise, admonish or guide, but to soothe and comfort as a companion to the ill or dying patient, rather than the authority. And in order to create a profession that is truly able to respond to the needs of a spiritually pluralistic society, professional healthcare chaplaincy must take note of the recent trends towards the disestablishment and individuation of spiritual identity and practice in society. Only if the profession is able to redefine itself and communicate effectively its relevance and ability to serve all patients, will it be able to overcome the prejudice that is exemplified by the National Secular Society 2009 criticism of the NHS Chaplaincy, that it is an archaic institution that only benefits a minority of patients and as such is not deserving of public funding that could be better spent on services with proven effects that benefit all patients (*The Telegraph* 2009).

Present and future practice

In the light of the above argument, and in considering recommendations for the future practice of healthcare chaplaincy, one of the areas requiring significant attention is the development of a solid methodology for spiritual care to the non-religious. Whilst even defining non-religious spiritual needs, let alone creating a new model of pastoral care to provide it, may be seen by some to be a daunting challenge, it can also be viewed as an opportunity to embrace and express the creativity of current practitioners and to become more multi-culturally literate, which will undoubtedly deepen and enrich the profession as a whole.

Theory

Through the multiplicity of definitions for the role of the chaplain, both spiritual and religious, one commonality is the role the chaplain plays in attending to existential crises. As a starting point for a theoretical model of non-religious care, this chapter points to an existing prototype, Frankl's logotherapy and existential analysis (Viktor Frankl Institut 2014). This model is a meaning-centred approach to applied psychotherapy that has its roots in philosophy and anthropology.

Logotherapy is of particular interest to the development of a theory and practice of non-religious chaplaincy because it exemplifies a secular practice that is clearly located in a spiritual care realm, and which can be differentiated from that of social work, for example. This is demonstrated by the consistent focus on, and use of, the term *human spirit* in a secular sense, as seen in this discussion of *Freedom of Will*:

> *Freedom is here defined as the space of shaping one's own life within the limits of the given possibilities. This freedom derives from the spiritual dimension of the person, which is understood as the essentially human realm, over and above the dimensions of body and of psyche. As spiritual persons, humans are not just reacting organisms but autonomous beings capable of actively shaping their lives. (Viktor Frankl Institut 2014)*

Logotherapy is founded on a set of six assumptions:

1. The human being is an entity consisting of body, mind and spirit.

2. Life has meaning under all circumstances, even the most miserable.

3. People have a will to find meaning.

4. People have freedom under all circumstances to activate the will to find meaning.

5. Life has a demand quality to which people must respond if decisions are to be meaningful.

6. The individual is unique.

(Viktor Frankl Institute of Logotherapy 2014)

These assumptions speak to some key principles of healthcare chaplaincy: the value and dignity of all people, the fostering of meaning-making, the potential of the human spirit to triumph in adversity. One of the key techniques of logotherapy that suggests its innate relevance to the practice of chaplaincy is the process of asking specific questions to help find and realise meaning. This conversation method originates with Socrates, who referred to it as a form of 'spiritual midwifery' (Viktor Frankl Institut 2014). This term is highly appropriate to the work of the healthcare chaplain, both in its suggestion of her role as an attendant to a major life event and transition, and because it alludes to supporting the person labouring, as opposed to the one labouring *for them*. One of the most important distinctions between ministry and chaplaincy is that in chaplaincy, as in logotherapy, one acts as the facilitator for the individual to find or create their own meaning, rather than suggesting an interpretation based on one's own doctrine or philosophy.

Practice

In terms of looking at specific practices that would complement a theoretical model of non-religious spiritual care, an examination of current resources is necessary. First, the Association of Professional Chaplains publishes a list of *Complementary Practices in Professional Chaplaincy* (Association of Professional Chaplains 2009). This list is described as a *work-in-progress* developed by the Commission on Quality in Pastoral Services, and contributions are invited of examples of practices that 'a chaplain could do within her/his setting of ministry and should be relevant to the mind/body/spirit continuum' (Association of Professional Chaplains 2009). The list contains a description alongside the purported benefits of each practice, together with research and resources for further exploration. Whilst some of these practices are exclusively religious, many of them would indeed be appropriate for consideration in compiling a tool box of non-religious spiritual care practices, including: anointing with oil; aromatherapy; art; breath work; chat rooms; chanting; confession; crystals; dream work; drumming; fasting; forgiveness; gratitude; guided imagery and visualisation; healing touch; humour; hypnosis; journalling; the contemplative practice of walking a labyrinth; laying on of hands; meditation; mindfulness; music; pets; play; poetry; qi gong; reflexology; reiki; relaxation and relaxation response; and spiritual direction.

A second resource worthy of mention is the *Alphabet of Spiritual Literacy* created by Frederic and Mary Ann Brussat (1998, pp.19–25), a compilation of 37 spiritual practices that are common in the world's religions. An example of how this practice might be adopted into a system of diagnosing and treating non-religious spiritual needs is contained in the Brussats' 'Spiritual Rx Prescriptions Chart' (2014).

Watson's Theory of Caring

Whilst designed as a theory of nursing, Watson's Theory of Caring has much to offer as a framework for the development of a curriculum for the pastoral practice of non-religious methodology for chaplaincy

(Watson 2005). The original theory, which was developed in 1979, was underpinned by ten 'carative' factors:

1. The formation of a humanistic-altruistic system of values.

2. The instillation of faith-hope.

3. The cultivation of sensitivity to one's self and to others.

4. The development of a helping-trust relationship.

5. The promotion and acceptance of the expression of positive and negative feelings.

6. The systematic use of the scientific problem-solving method for decision making.

7. The promotion of interpersonal teaching-learning.

8. The provision for a supportive, protective, and/or corrective mental, physical, sociocultural and spiritual environment.

9. Assistance with the gratification of human needs.

10. The allowance for existential-phenomenological forces.

(Rosenberg 2006, p.53; see also Watson 1994)

This original theory evolved into the *Clinical Caritas Processes* (Watson 2008). *Caritas* is used in the sense of the Christian theological virtue of *agape*. These processes seem well suited upon which to base a new system of competencies for training and evaluation of chaplains as skilled providers of non-religious spiritual care:

- practice of loving–kindness and equanimity within the context of caring consciousness

- being authentically present, and enabling and sustaining the deep belief system and subjective life world of self and one-being-cared-for

- cultivation of one's own spiritual practices and transpersonal self, going beyond the ego self

- developing and sustaining a helping–trusting, authentic caring relationship

- being present to, and supportive of, the expression of positive and negative feelings as a connection with deeper spirit of self and the one-being-cared-for

- creative use of self and all ways of knowing as part of the caring process; to engage in the artistry of caring–healing practices

- engaging in genuine teaching–learning experience that attends to unity of being and meaning, attempting to stay within other's frame of reference

- creating healing environment at all levels (physical as well as non-physical), subtle environment of energy and consciousness, whereby wholeness, beauty, comfort, dignity, and peace are potentiated

- assisting with basic needs, with an intentional caring consciousness, administering 'human care essentials', which potentiate alignment of mind–body–spirit, wholeness, and unity of being in all aspects of care; tending to both embodied spirit and evolving spiritual emergence

- opening and attending to spiritual-mysterious and existential dimensions of one's own life–death; soul care for self and the one-being-cared-for.

(Foster 2007)

The epistemological and philosophical basis of the model helps to distinguish the practice from psycho-social disciplines by firmly rooting it in the transcendental:

Levinas' ethical starting point, which locates itself within a universal field of infinite love, as the primordial source for sustaining our humanity and as the source for all human evolution. Therefore, a metaphysical relationship between our physical-scientific world and the universal infinity of the evolving human consciousness is re-established. (Watson 2005, p.304)

This model is worthy of further consideration by those designing the future curriculum of healthcare chaplaincy for another reason. Coming as it does from the discipline of nursing, this model has been put into practice in the hospital setting, which has entailed the evolution and definition of a methodology of assessment and interventions that can be recorded in clinical documentation. When a Chicago hospital implemented this practice, it was deemed that new terminology would be required in order to facilitate clinical documentation. The process led to the creation of a new nursing diagnosis designed to help clinicians accurately document a specific problem, 'Compromised Human Dignity' (Rosenberg 2006). Future research might investigate how this model compares with current tools of spiritual assessment and documentation utilised by pastoral care practitioners at present and what this approach might have to offer to the profession.

In conclusion, rigorous self-reflection will be essential for the development of a new model of healthcare chaplaincy in a pluralistic society. In finding the courage to be unafraid to question or even throw away the mould and to challenge the established ways of doing things, new possibilities are invited:

Tom Beaudoin, expresses this sentiment exquisitely:

> *Foucauldian thought forces us to begin to confront the vertigo of the radically historical character of our identities. The purpose of this logic is twofold: first, to refuse the contingent and historical limits on what we can be, limits that are reinforced by institutions and traditions that benefit from fixing one historical configuration of the self as the eternal or natural self; and second, to create new ways of practicing ourselves, of more varied and creative freedoms in our present. (Beaudoin 2008)*

The profession and the people it seeks to care for will be best served by the perception of this situation as an opportunity, rather than a threat. It is an opportunity to design a truly inclusive practice of Spiritual Care that will be nurturing to all.

CHAPTER 8

Developing a Model of Chaplaincy through the Translation of Nursing Theory

Debbie Hodge

Introduction

This chapter explores how healthcare chaplaincy can develop models of practice in dialogue with nursing theory and practice. It draws on both the author's own experience of the transition from nursing to chaplaincy, and on systematic reflection shared with a reflective-practice group of other chaplains. The model that emerges was developed in dialogue with a chaplaincy collaborative, and is set within the context of contemporary healthcare chaplaincy, and the practical and political issues that arises for chaplains. At the heart of the model is an approach characterised by encounter, relationship and transaction, which maintains the value of the human interaction between chaplain and patient, carer or staff member; and which enables them to develop and deploy a shared 'tool box' of approaches to spiritual and human need.

The landscape

The work of the chaplain in the modern NHS is very different to the historic picture of the Anglican cleric described by Chris Swift (2009, Chapter 1). Today in the NHS, chaplains are employees in an environment that is secular in nature yet working with, through and for individuals with a wide range of cultural, religious and spiritual backgrounds and traditions.

Within this environment the chaplain, along with all healthcare professionals, needs to be able to account for the work they do. The minimum data-set was established in November 2005, providing chaplains with a mechanism to detail how they spent their time, and to show, at least, in terms of number of hours, who they were engaging with, even if outcomes of that activity were not measured directly (on the minimum data-set, see Chapter 5).

Questions over evidence-based practice, efficacy of the service offered, along with budget revisions mean that chaplains in all areas of the NHS have to be able to describe the 'how' and the 'what' of their actions and to follow up the interventions with evaluation that details their contribution to health outcomes. Today they need to address such questions as: What contribution do they make to the patient experience? What were the immediate and longer term effects on health outcomes? How did their intervention supplement or support that of other healthcare professionals?

The key changes in the NHS in England over the last ten years have also marked out the territory for chaplains. For example, the NHS Constitution (Department of Health 2013) used the word 'compassion' as a key descriptor of the service, and this was taken up by nursing in the form of the '6Cs for Nursing', namely: care; compassion; competence; communication; courage; and commitment (Department of Health 2012).

For chaplains, however, 'compassion' is a tangible demonstration arising from their faith tradition, the outworking of theological integration and the pastoral expedient. Harrison in his article 'Exploring the relationship between the understandings and practices of compassion in healthcare chaplaincy and other healthcare contexts' noted that 'for the chaplain there is relevance to a healthcare system that asserts compassion as a value, but that "system" may not be aware that the chaplain draws on a "rich source of compassion" because of their faith' (Harrison 2012, p.54).

The Equality Act 2010, the Health and Social Care Act (2012), the Francis report[1] (February 2013) and the End of Life Care Alliance's work have all helped shape the modern NHS. Add to this ever-increasing cultural diversity, the 'Prevent Strategy', higher patient/ client expectations, developments in pharmaceuticals and surgical intervention, increasing financial pressure and the need for each profession in the health system to mark their territory – makes for a very complex agenda for chaplaincy to navigate.

Insight from the history of nursing

In the 1970s and 1980s the same sort of challenges faced nursing, as the profession faced the question: What do nurses do? This led to key developments in nursing, and to a collection of work on the theory of nursing – an attempt to provide a model or framework that would enable others to appreciate what approach the nurse was taking and the outcomes of care interventions. Schober (in Hinchliff, Norman and Schober 1989, p.172) noted that nursing theory could contribute towards resolving ambiguity (in nursing) by showing what is happening and serving as a predictor of nursing actions (and outcomes).

The development of nursing theory began with the question: What is nursing? This led to wider debate on what was the 'focus' of nursing action. The 'person' was identified as the focus – whether called client or patient, and nursing action was the 'activity' with an individual.

Fitzpatrick and Whall (1989) conducted an analysis of the emerging nursing theories and noted that the conceptual models contributed significantly to the development of nursing as a profession with an emerging body of knowledge that was specific to that discipline. There was, however, an omission – spiritual care was not an explicit focus, although for some (reaching back to Nightingale) there was a religious element. For those in the nursing profession at this time much of what was 'done' was seen as 'common sense' but was in fact the learnt art of nursing developed from experience, a demonstration of the 'novice to expert' progression identified by Benner (1982).

Within nursing theories key building blocks were described that related to the 'person' who was the focus of care, 'nursing' – the actions of that care, 'health' and the 'environment'. It was not until 1998 that the three primary elements of the International Classification for Nursing Practice (ICNP) were described as: (i) nursing phenomena, i.e. the focus of nursing, sometimes referred to as nursing diagnosis; (ii) nursing interventions, i.e. the actions or activities nurses perform; and (iii) nursing outcomes, i.e. the results of nurses' actions in terms of change in the focus at a specific time.

Florence Nightingale described the individual as having physical, intellectual, emotional, social and spiritual components. She also espoused the principle that all persons are equal. For her, health was an 'additive process', the combined results of environment (the physical elements external to the patient), physical and psychological factors. To be well was to be able to use every power one had. Nursing was described in religious terms: 'Service to God in the relief of man' (Nightingale 1858), and, 'to put the patient in the best condition for nature to act upon him' (Nightingale 1859/1969, p.133). These descriptors were based on her experience and observations.

It was Virginia Henderson (1991) who described a 'patient centred' approach to nursing. For her the individual is a biological being, in whom mind and body are inseparable. He/she requires food, shelter, communication, the company of loved ones, the opportunity to learn, work, play and worship; and to be healthy is to have the ability to function independently. The action of the nurse is 'to assist the patient – sick or well, in performance of those activities that he/she would perform unaided, and to gain independence'. The environment was not well defined.

For Imogen King the individual is seen as an open system interacting with the environment. Engaging individual, interpersonal and community systems that are dynamic and interacting, health is a dynamic life experience that implies continuous adjustment to stressors in the internal and external environment through optimum use of one's resources to achieve maximum potential for daily living (King 1981, p.5). Nursing aims 'to help individuals maintain their health so that they can function in their roles' (King 1981, pp.4–5). It is in the interpersonal system nurse–client, that the traditional steps of the nursing process are carried out. From this perspective, environment is an open system with permeable boundaries permitting an exchange of matter, energy and information with human beings. It was King who demonstrated the interrelational nature of the person in the context of family/friends, community and ultimately the world; and thus the relational nature of nursing. This was the model that I used to inform my practice as a nurse, and it was from this basis that I developed my ways of describing the individual, health, nursing and environment.

The key question: What do chaplains do, and can nursing theory inform the discussion?

To explore this question further, I engaged with a group of chaplains – the South West Midlands Collaborative – who spent time reflecting on their everyday practice and discerning a pathway that began to paint a picture of activity and outcome. The group had been meeting since the introduction of Chaplaincy Collaboratives in the 'Caring for the Spirit' project (2003). In their meetings there was an established pattern of reflective practice, usually built around a 'case study' or 'critical incident'.

The request for facilitation to help them discern a way of understanding what they did had arisen out of conversations with some chaplains in the local area, and work previously shared in answering the question 'What do chaplains need to know?' in a multi-faith context. This particular piece of work was based on Carper's work on 'patterns of knowing' (1978), in which she described how nursing was a practice discipline based on scientific, ethical and personal knowledge melded together into the art of nursing through the relationship of the nurse with the patient and their family/carers.

The aim of the reflection with the collaborative was to discern how the ideas on the development of nursing theory might serve to help chaplains to develop a framework that could:

1. enable other healthcare professionals to understand what chaplains do

2. contribute towards resolving ambiguity (in chaplaincy) by showing what is happening

3. serve as a predictor of chaplaincy action (and outcomes).

The process

The reflective practice group

As the collaborative had been meeting for reflective practice sessions for a while, ground rules had been established. Those principles were adopted for this work, and included confidentiality, one person speaking at a time, the shared belief that no comment is too small, no question too big to be shared and respect for all in the group. Such reflective practice is the self-conscious discipline of critically interpreting and understanding experience through the active engagement with what we know of others, the particular context and ourselves; and seeing this as key in the development of the practical knowledge of chaplaincy (Cobb 2005, pp.29, 30). It is used by all healthcare professionals and can serve to develop their practice and improve patient care/outcomes. It is also a key component in building research awareness.

For chaplains there is an added layer in the reflection process – the theological element. This is essential for the chaplain as it supports the underpinning structures for their ways of being and the values they place on life, health and humanity. It also informs their ethical and moral thinking (see UK Board of Healthcare Chaplaincy 2009, Capabilities 4.1 and 4.2).

Meetings were held approximately every three months and in between meetings homework was set. This related to the areas under discussion for the session and to issues to be covered in the next session. Each meeting lasted about an hour and a half.

Reflective conversations

In exploring the four key building blocks of person, health, chaplaincy and environment (adapted from King's approach to nursing discussed earlier), the chaplains of the collaborative offered the following definitional terms:

- Person, unique human being, made in God's image, connected to family, friends, community and God, sum of body, mind and spirit, 'personhood' needing love and belongingness.

- Health/healing, not about cure, the integration of body, mind and spirit, death is the ultimate healing, being whole, wholeness, healing achievable by all, whose view is the 'right view'?,[2] well staff means well patients.

- Chaplaincy, holistic compassion, vulnerability, acceptance, forgiveness, empathy stillness and silence, 'soaking up' or 'holding' situations, emotions and spiritual distress, presence – being present, a 'representative' of something, 'other', making the 'other' visible, bridge builder, safety net.

- Environment, sacred space, holy ground, illness had made the familiar landscape that was the patient into an alien one, fear of the environment, context, who owned the 'environment'?, alienation, welcoming the stranger, radical hospitality, asylum.

These responses had clear resonance with nursing aims, for example, to enable the patient to be independent, and return to role function; and with the view that there is no compulsion to 'fix'. This resonance is reflected in the language, which speaks of 'presence', 'holding', being a 'safety net'. But it also suggests even less of an activist agenda amongst chaplains, in comparison with nurses. There was also a distinctiveness in the views on health – the chaplains quickly replaced 'health' with 'healing', stating that 'healing was achievable by all'. They also articulated the difference between healing and cure.

The chaplains also acknowledged that they worked in three paradigms – pastoral, spiritual and religious, although for many in society religion has little meaning,[3] and like nurses with three sets of people, patients, staff and friends/relatives.

It became apparent that these descriptions, while at the heart of their everyday work, were linked to the deeply held and sustaining narrative of their faith and personal spirituality, which was the meta-narrative of the Christian gospel (the group was for the most part Christian with occasional attendance of the Muslim chaplain). The responses also gave weight to the motivation, or drivers, for the work chaplains do – a calling or vocation from God, rooted in God's love and grace (Ephesians 5:15–17).

Having identified the building blocks the group began to explore the nature of the work that they did with individuals and groups and how they might describe the phases of their work.

Encounter

The initial phase of chaplaincy was described as 'encounter'. This phase was described as the 'testing out' of the situation and the people involved, and imaged as a butterfly 'extending its proboscis and sensing the situation' or 'a snake tasting the air with a flicking tongue'. Such images acted as descriptions of 'sensing the situation – soaking up the atmosphere'. The key need from the chaplain was 'making sense of the situation'.

The chaplains in the group noted that they were 'Asking myself – why am I here, what's the story?' 'Seeking permission – am I welcome here, am I needed here?' All agreed that the encounter 'Involves a greeting – and the look on your face and the look in your eyes' is key to establishing a rapport.

The language used in this section is in part almost poetic, yet also practical – 'What is going on here?' 'What's the story?' In most other professions the initial encounter starts with some form of greeting – so too in the chaplaincy world. But the greeting from the chaplain is also conveying a question – a seeking of permission, and is linked with the 'building block' statements, as the response to the greeting will convey much about the situation or 'story' and the individuals concerned.

Relationship

This initial 'encounter' provides the bedrock of the chaplains' work and leads to a 'relationship'. It is in this phase that the work on discerning dis-ease is centred, or, using the language of the NHS, where an assessment is made of pastoral, spiritual and religious needs.

The group's reflection included statements such as: 'We work in a world of mystery, approach things through allegory and metaphor – able to say hard things and ask hard questions'; 'We pick up on language – word and symbol – touching on a common language'; 'Acknowledge Spiritual distress – in all its forms – but what is behind it?'. They also spoke of 'Reaching out on a human basis'; and of how this work 'Involves advocacy'.

The relationship can be built in five minutes and in some cases may be as short as that – or can last for months – but in that relationship many issues are explored and questions raised for and in the chaplain as well as the 'patient'; and the patient may begin to express something of their 'need'. As Shelly notes 'spiritual needs may seem elusive' (2000, p.30) and, while those needs may be observed, they can be hard to pin down or measure. The words the chaplains used when identifying different manifestations of spiritual distress were many and varied and included guilt, hatred, anger, isolation, fear, loneliness, anxiety, pain, tears and silence.

The group also discerned that what they were offering, through their 'presence' and 'holding' of the situation, was 'fragile hope' and 'compassion'. Ricoeur calls hope a 'passion for the possible', which asserts meaning and value over chaos and destruction (Ricoeur 1995, in Reynolds 2008, p.141), and is seen by Farley as 'an existential refusal of the denomination of the Tragic' (Reynolds 2008, p.142). These descriptors again point to the sustaining metanarrative of the Christian gospel.

The two stories that follow serve to elucidate the building of relationship; the first is from a chaplain who was asked to visit a patient and, after the greeting and seeking permission to be there, the deep truth emerged. In the second there is a developing relationship that allows the exploration of feelings and the use of story to give a different perspective.

STORY 1. LONELINESS

After a few moments, the patient said 'my daughter hasn't spoken to me since I had the diagnosis of cancer'.

STORY 2. ON THE EDGE

A lady with long-standing depression and low self-esteem struggles with her faith, God being distant and not hearing her cries. She has been experiencing herself as on the margins, an outcast – which is a totally negative image. During guided meditation we explored life on the margins and were brought to reflect upon the margins of the fields left uncultivated for the poor to eat – spoken of in Leviticus and by Jesus. In the margins there is rubbish, excrement, vermin and pests and wild animals, yet also food to be shared with the poor, outcast and lost. If this lady finds herself placed in the margins then it can be seen as positive, as a God-given role, living with the s**t, yet being able to give life through food and company to the poor and the outcast. She found it a profoundly helpful picture and it has been a key part of her recovery – namely finding God in her experience of depression and being an outcast. Perhaps finding meaning in a place with no meaning.

As indicated previously, it is in the relationship phase that the spiritual, pastoral and religious needs are discerned. This gives rise to the question of how chaplains do ascertain spiritual needs and discern dis-ease? The question of spiritual assessment has been, and continues to be, debated by nurses. However, spiritual assessment has been recognised as a distinct role of healthcare chaplains by the WHO for over a decade (Cobb *et al.* 2012). In general, assessment is the taking of some kind of measurement and 'assessing' those findings against 'average' figures. For example, a nurse will take the patient's blood pressure and will compare the measurement with what is 'normal' and then take appropriate action.

There are a variety of 'spiritual assessment tools', some of which are used by nurses and other healthcare professionals to give a 'spiritual or religious history'. One such is the HOPE tool (Anandarajah and Hight 2001). This is concerned with discerning: H – sources of hope, meaning, comfort, strength, peace, love and connection; O – organised religion; P – personal spirituality/practices; E – effects on medical care and end-of-life issues. Other models include those known as FICA (F – Faith or belief; I – Importance and Influence, C – Community, A – Address needs) (Puchalski and Romer 2000) and FACT (F – Faith (and/or Beliefs, Spiritual Practices; A – Active and/or Availability, Accessibility, Applicability; C – Coping and/or Comfort; Conflict and/or Concern; T – Treatment Plan) (LaRocca-Pitts 2012). When it comes to assessing spiritual need there is no set 'norm' against which to measure so that action can be planned. The assessment of pastoral, spiritual (and religious) needs can be seen in the light of the 'relationship' in which the key essence of need may be expressed.

What the chaplains from the collaborative were able to discuss was not just the kind of conversations they had – which at times would have explored issues in HOPE, FICA and FACT, with perhaps a nuance of language, but more about the attention they gave to the patient's responses. How chaplains use the responses that patients offer and where, through the building of a relationship of trust, that leads to is illustrated in the following two stories.

STORY 3. SITTING ON GRANDMA'S KNEE

Billy is a tall young man in the local psychiatric unit. He has at times become very agitated and has the potential to become physically abusive. When these episodes occur standard practice leads to Billy being isolated. Billy finds these episodes tiring and he wants them to stop. The chaplain had been visiting regularly and Billy enjoyed the chaplain's visits. One day the chaplain asked, 'Can you tell me about a time when you felt safe and comforted?' Billy smiles – 'When I was with my grandma – I would sit on her knee and she would sing Kumbaya.' He begins to sing. His whole demeanour changes, the tightness goes from his jaw and there is a faint smile on his lips. He finishes the song and all is quiet.

STORY 4. CAN WE BUY A YELLOW T-SHIRT?

Kathy had been in hospital for eight months. She was now in the rehabilitation unit and preparing to go home. Following a bone marrow transplant, complications had developed and, after spells in the intensive care unit and the palliative care ward, she was at last ready to go home. But she hadn't anything to wear, and she didn't want her clothes from home as they would not fit. 'Would not fit?' the chaplain echoed. 'Will they not fit who you are now?' In conversation with the staff, the chaplain was able to share this concern of Kathy's and the next outing from the unit was not just to the coffee shop, but was a trip to River Island to find a yellow T-shirt and a pair of skinny jeans. When her husband and children arrived a few days later there was much chat about the new clothes – and the outing to get them. Kathy told the chaplain that she had heard the words she had been waiting for from her husband – 'You are you again!'

In story three, the question asked by the chaplain was 'When did you feel safe?', rather than 'What is making you frightened?' By exploring from a different view point and seeking something different or 'other' from the client, the chaplain was able to bring about a different resolution. In discussion with the staff an alternative care plan was put in place. At the first signs of agitation someone would go and sit with Billy and sing Kumbaya. All the staff learnt the song, and Billy's episodes of fear and panic were managed in a very different way.

In story four the conversation with the staff gave the chaplain the opportunity to share, not just the practical aspect of Kathy's lack of clothes that fitted, but what that represented. Kathy's treatment and care had been invasive and she felt she had lost who she was through that invasive care. The yellow T-shirt and the skinny jeans were her way of reclaiming her identity. Would it have been easier for the staff to ask her husband to buy the clothes and bring them in? Yes – but that would have not given Kathy back the control she had lost, even in what some might see as the small thing of choosing what clothes to wear.

Fear and anxiety, problems of self-image, pain, concern, cancer, surgery, are all words that to some may mean a 'diagnosis', or a 'label', and are the currency of specific healthcare professionals, as they seek to mark their territory and identify the unique currency of their work. Yet for the chaplains engaged in this particular set of conversations, these were the very words that led to something deeper, something that was affecting the soul (and therefore the mind and body). The words were 'cues into' deeper needs and understanding. It was the recognition that the words the patient was using were the only words they had to explain something more. It was the chaplain who could, in the safe place they had created and through skilled communication, enable the patient to articulate those things that seemed beyond words. Clayton (2013) describes such a situation, in which the space was created for a family to say goodbye to their dying baby. Citing the work of Dennis Potter he notes that the creation of that space had given them an opportunity to stand at the 'cauldron of the actual minute' and allow tumultuous emotions to bubble up.

While there are useful tools for taking a spiritual and religious history that enable chaplains (and others) to make a spiritual or religious needs assessment, they are of little use unless some form of action occurs. And, while it may be possible to meet religious needs and provide rituals (e.g. time for prayer, holy communion), and maintain the spiritual connection with the local faith community through visits by the local faith leaders, the risk remains that deeper religious and spiritual needs of faith in the face of diagnosis or death may go unrecognised. The craft and practice of the chaplain will allow for those needs to be expressed through the developing relationship, which allows for sacred space (the environment) to be created in which needs can be expressed and then met.

In the examples given, it was the skill of the chaplain in using the patients' own words that led to a different kind of question or conversation; and to action to meet deep-felt needs. As the stories illustrate the actions were not extravagant, although did need a bit of planning!

Sharing the tool box transaction

In chaplaincy it is acknowledged that each person involved in the encounter has much to share in the meeting of pastoral, spiritual and religious needs. A patient doesn't leave their life experience at the door of the hospital, nor do they leave behind everything in the world they usually inhabit. The chaplain has a tool box of knowledge, skills, rituals and life and chaplaincy experience to share with the patient; and the patient has their tool box too.

When asked what would be found in their tool box the chaplains from the collaborative noted the following: faith, hope, love, openness, vulnerability, self-awareness, presence, humility, compassion, self and discernment, and saw these as personal attributes. Their tool box also included the Bible, prayer, reflection, language, symbolic action, priestly role, sacrament and being commissioned by God.

The contents described, once again linked back to their personal faith and the meta-narrative of the Christian gospel (note – much of the content would also be found in the tool boxes of those of faiths and beliefs other than Christianity). The tool box of the patient, built over time, will contain their resources and the learning that they have gathered, lived through and developed. When both boxes are opened and the sharing begins there can be those moments of deep connection that enhance the experience and provide a reconnection for the patient that mitigates their spiritual or religious distress.

When there is that 'connection' something is 'transacted'. There is a shift in thinking, feeling, being, that has effects on the patient and the chaplain. Transaction occurs because the process is not one way: working with a patient has an effect on the chaplain. The chaplains noted that this is perhaps the hardest part of the process to discern, for in it all there is at work greater forces than they can know or describe. The fruit of this work however is seen in the outcomes.

Outcomes and reflection

All outcomes of pastoral, spiritual and religious care need describing and translating. They may be described in religious language, or in spiritual or pastoral language – but that may not be understood by the patient or other healthcare professionals. The group discovered that, while they had made a note that the patient said 'they were more peaceful' or that it was 'good to talk things through', the chaplain had not been going back to see if the peace lasted (e.g. did the patient sleep better), or if talking things through had reduced anxiety (e.g. was the patient happier to talk about what had brought them to hospital with the other members of the caring team).

The identification of the outcomes of pastoral, spiritual and religious care is of little consequence in the wider picture of health if they are not evaluated and communicated. Once identified the 'outcomes' are reflected on and their impact established for patient, chaplain, other members of the caring team, and the planned care of that patient.

Gathering the threads

As a former nurse I was used to thinking in the four realms – person, health, nursing and environment, and working with a model of nursing which closely related to that of King (1981). On moving into Christian ministry and then to healthcare chaplaincy, I began to explore how chaplaincy might look if the same principles were applied. The incident that provoked these thoughts came from journeying with a patient throughout their last stay in hospital, which lasted four months. I had been called to the intensive care unit to visit a patient who was having difficulty in discerning her way forward having been given some stark information regarding her breathing and the implications of further intervention to support that. Following this particular individual and supporting her through both the trauma of refusing intervention for her breathing problems, to her move to palliative care, then on to the rehabilitation unit and home, I had the opportunity to reflect on my transition from nurse to chaplain alongside the changes in my approach to how I ordered my ways of working.

As a chaplain, my philosophical framework has shifted from one where my key motivation was to enable the patient to become independent (after Henderson 1991) or support the continuous adjustment to internal and external stressors so that the individual may achieve their maximum potential (after King 1981), to one that was motivated by my belief that everyone was entitled to have 'life in all abundance' (Gospel of St John, Chapter 10, Verse 10). My reference now is theological and spiritual, not just physiological, sociological or psychological. Tournier (1986 p.50), following his encounter with a doctor in Japan, wrote 'I realise that in every sick person there is not only a psychological perspective but also a spiritual one; and that there is a reciprocal relationship, as there is between body and soul, between the physical – the domain of classical medicine – and the propositions of religion'.

Those key building blocks from a theological, spiritual and philosophical understanding have reshaped my view of patient, health, chaplaincy and environment. The individual is now seen as a unique unity with physiological, psychological, sociological and spiritual (and religious) elements, worthy of empathy, respect and care: with the right to life in all abundance. Health has become the integration of body, mind and spirit. This has some resonance with my early work as a nurse on taking the patient's view of their health. It was Dr Calman (as Chief Medical Officer) who quoted a patient as saying 'health – it's just about getting through my day'. Chaplaincy is seen as pertaining to the individual and the service that enables the individual, well or sick, to integrate body, mind and spirit, and to find meaning in the chaos of illness, where this is enacted in an environment that facilitates the safe space to enable the work of chaplaincy to be done.

In my nursing career I used the nursing process (based on the problem solving cycle of assess, plan, implement and evaluate) to order my work. As a chaplain the basic framework is still there but now the language has changed. In the light of the reflective conversations with the collaborative, I now view assessment as being built up from meeting the patient (the 'encounter') and developing a 'relationship' that allows spiritual needs to emerge before engaging in ways to support the meeting of those needs (the 'transaction' involving patient, chaplain and others). Vital in this model is evaluating what difference has been made and reflecting on that to discern further ways of supporting the individual and the ongoing learning for future situations.

Placing the described elements in the problem solving cycle there is a correlation between the way I worked as a nurse and the way I work as a chaplain. This is a key development, enabling chaplains to speak into the nursing world and nurses to understand that chaplains also follow a process that can be explained!

Nursing	Problem Solving	Chaplaincy
Assessment	Assess	Encounter
↓	↓	↓
Identify need	Plan	Relationship
↓	↓	↓
Plan and implement	Implement	Transaction
↓	↓	↓
Evaluate	Evaluate	Outcomes and Reflection

**Figure 8.1 The process of chaplaincy in the
context of the nursing process**

Figure 8.1 shows the process of chaplaincy in the context of the nursing process. The linear representation, however, when worked out in practice, becomes spiral in nature – in that the aspects of the process may be revisited over time and the process with one particular individual or encounter/action provides the antecedents for the next encounter.

Figure 8.2 puts the information into that format.

This locates: the terms that chaplains use to describe ways of 'being' and 'doing' that enable them to gain a sense of the situation (like a butterfly sensing the atmosphere or a snake using its tongue to sense meaning); the developing relationship linked to 'sacred space'; and the sense of safety that 'asylum' brings. It further acknowledges that patients/clients have personal and spiritual resources, as well as the chaplain (sharing tool boxes), that play a significant part in meeting spiritual needs and contributing to health outcomes. The outlined process of chaplaincy process linked to the key building blocks provides a framework that enables chaplains to articulate what they do, in words and actions. The key in all this is the use of the patients' responses.

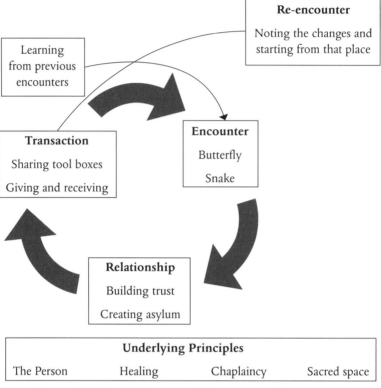

Figure 8.2 The spiral nature of the process of chaplaincy

Was the question answered?

The framework does give a way of sharing the 'what' and 'how' of chaplaincy and resolving ambiguity in chaplaincy by showing what is happening. The question remaining is 'Can it serve as a predictor of chaplaincy actions and outcomes?' I would argue that the model provides reliable foundations for future action, as well as room to continuously revisit and develop those foundations. Building a repertoire of encounters and relationships, together with a tool box of approaches to mutual spiritual care within the relationships is, in one sense, predictive. It develops the chaplain's confidence in the human interaction of spiritual care. But this approach is not prescriptive and nor can it be. Given the difficulty of articulating health outcomes in the languages of theology, religion, philosophy or spirituality, and the need for a patient-centred approach that works with his language of spiritual care, the chaplain needs space to be flexible, responsive and imaginative in the human encounters and relationships at the heart of healthcare chaplaincy. The process of chaplaincy outlined here offers this, while underpinning it with an evidence base of developing practice.

Notes

1. The final report of The Mid Staffordshire NHS Foundation Trust Public Inquiry (2013), chaired by Robert Francis QC.
2. Moltmann (1985) cautioned that 'the ideas of "health" may not be necessarily "healthy", supporting comments that the person's view of health for them may not be "healthy", leading to questions of whose health is it?'
3. In the 2011 Census for England and Wales, 59.3 per cent of the usual resident population (33.2 million people) identified as Christian. Muslims made up the second largest religious group, with 4.8 per cent of the population (2.7 million people). A quarter of the population (14.1 million people) reported they had no religion.

REFERENCES

Legislation and case law

Prison Act 1952.

Prison Ministers Act 1863.

The Criminal Justice Act 1991.

Data Protection Act 1998.

Article 9 of the European Convention of Human Rights.

Article 14 of the European Convention of Human Rights.

Constitution of the World Health Organization, opened for signature 22 July 1946, 62 Stat. 2769, 14 U.N.T.S. 185.

Lithgow v UK 1986 3 EHRR 329.

X v UK (1983) 5 EHRR 289.

Books and journal articles

Abbott, A. (1988) *The System Of Professions: An Essay on the Division of Expert Labor.* Chicago, IL: University of Chicago Press.

ACLU (2008) 'ACLU sues to protect marriages threatened by recent court decision.' Available at: www.aclu.org/religion-belief/aclu-sues-protect-marriages-threatened-recent-court-decision (accessed 19 February 2015).

ACLU (2014) 'The ACLU and freedom of religion and belief.' Available at: www.aclu.org/religion-belief-workshop/aclu-and-freedom-religion-and-belief (accessed 19 February 2015).

AHPCC (2013) 'Future of chaplaincy workshop notes.' Available at: www.ahpcc.org.uk//study-policy-2/the-future-of-chaplaincy/ (accessed 24 May 2015).

Anandarajah, G. and Hight, E. (2001) 'Spirituality and medical practice: Using the HOPE questions as a practical tool for spiritual assessment.' *American Family Physician 63,* 1, 81–88.

Anderson, R.G. (2004) 'The Search for Spiritual/Cultural Competency in Chaplaincy Practice: Five Steps that Mark the Path.' In R.G. Anderson and M.A. Fukuyama (eds) *Ministry in the Spiritual and Cultural Diversity of Health Care: Increasing the Competency of Chaplains.* Binghamton, NY: The Haworth Press.

Association of Hospice and Palliative Care Chaplains (2005) 'Health care chaplaincy: Code of conduct.' Inverness, UK: Association of Hospice and Palliative Care Chaplains.

Association of Professional Chaplains (2009) 'Complementary spiritual practices in professional chaplaincy.' Available at: www.professionalchaplains.org/files/resources/reading_room/complementary_spiritual_practices.pdf (accessed 19 February 2015).

Association of Professional Chaplains, Association for Clinical Pastoral Education, Canadian Association for Pastoral Practice and Education, National Association of Catholic Chaplains and National Association of Jewish Chaplains (2001) 'A White Paper. Professional chaplaincy: Its role and importance in healthcare.' *Journal of Pastoral Care 55,* 1, 81–97.

Baldacchino, D. and Draper, P. (2001) 'Spiritual coping strategies: A review of the nursing research literature.' *Journal of Advanced Nursing 34,* 6, 833–841.

Basdevant-Gaudemet, B. (2005) 'State and Church in France.' In G. Robbers (ed.) *State and Church in the European Union* (second edition). Baden-Baden, Germany: European Consortium for State and Church Research.

Beauchamp, T.L. and Childress, J.F. (1994) *Principles of Biomedical Ethics* (fourth edition). Oxford, UK and New York: Oxford University Press.

Beaudoin, T. (2008) Witness to Dispossession: The Vocation of a Postmodern Theologian. Maryknoll, New York: Orbis Books.

Beckford, J.A. and Gilliat, S. (1996) 'The Church of England and other faiths in a multi-faith society.' Warwick, UK: University of Warwick, Department of Sociology.

Beckford, J. and Gilliat, S. (1998) *Religion in Prison: Equal Rites in a Multi-Faith Society*. Cambridge, UK: Cambridge University Press.

Benner, P. (1982) 'From novice to expert.' *The American Journal of Nursing 82*, 3, 402.

Berlinger, N. (2004) 'Spirituality and medicine: Idiot-proofing the discourse.' *Journal of Medicine and Philosophy 29*, 6, 681–695.

Bourdieu, P. (1986) 'The Forms of Capital.' In J.E. Richardson (ed.) *Handbook of Theory and Research for the Sociology of Education*. New York: Greenwood Press.

Brassey, P.D. (2009) 'Eliminate endorsement.' *PlainViews: An E-Newsletter for Chaplains and Other Spiritual Care Providers*.

Brussat, F. and Brussat, M. (1998) *Spiritual Literacy: Reading the Sacred in Everyday Life.* New York: Touchstone.

Brussat, F. and Brussat, M. (2014) 'Spiritual Rx prescriptions chart.' Available at: www.spiritualityandpractice.com/practices/chart.php (accessed 19 February 2015).

Buzan, B., Waever, O. and de Wilde, J. (1998) *Security: A New Framework for Analysis*. London: Lynne Rienner.

Cadge, W. (2012) Paging God: *Religion in the Halls of Medicine*. Chicago: The University of Chicago Press.

Carper, B. (1978) 'Fundamental patterns of knowing in nursing.' *Advances in Nursing Science 1*, 1, 13–23.

Carr, W. (2001) 'Spirituality and Religion: Chaplaincy in Context.' In H. Orchard (ed.) *Spirituality in Health Care Contexts*. London: Jessica Kingsley Publishers.

Clayton, M. (2013) 'Contemplative chaplaincy? A view from a children's hospice.' *Practical Theology 6*, 1, 35–50.

Cobb, M. (2005) *The Hospital Chaplain's Handbook*. Norwich, UK: Canterbury Press.

Cobb, M., Puchalski, C. and Rumbold, B. (eds) (2012) *The Oxford Text Book of Spiritual Health*. Oxford, UK: Oxford University Press.

Coleman, P.G., Ivani-Chalian, C. and Robinson, M. (2004) 'Religious attitudes among British older people: Stability and change in a 20-year longitudinal study.' *Ageing and Society 24*, 2, 167–188.

Craddock Lee, S.J. (2002) 'In a secular spirit: Strategies of clinical pastoral education.' *Health Care Analysis 10*, 339–356.

Cramer, E. and Tenzek, K.E. (2012) 'The chaplain profession from the employer perspective: An analysis of hospice chaplain job advertisements.' *Journal of Health Care Chaplaincy 18*, 133–150.

Curlin, F.A., Lantos, J.D., Roach, C.J., Sellergren, S.A. and Chin, M.H. (2005) 'Religious characteristics of U.S. physicians: A national survey.' *Journal of General Internal Medicine 20*, 7, 629–634.

Davie, G. (1990) 'Believing without belonging.' *Social Compass 37*, 455–469.

Department of Health (2001) 'Your guide to the NHS: Getting the most from your National Health Service.' London: Department of Health.

Department of Health (2003) 'NHS chaplaincy: Meeting the religious and spiritual needs of patients and staff.' London: Department of Health.

Department of Health (2012) 'NHS Commissioning Board – Compassion in practice.' London: Department of Health.

Department of Health (2013) 'The NHS constitution of England.' London: Department of Health.

Doe, N. (2002) *The Law of the Church in Wales*. Cardiff, UK: University of Wales Press.

Doe, N. and Payne, H. (2003) *Public Health and the limits of religions freedom*. Paper submitted for the European-American Law and Religion Consortium, Budapest, December.

Durkheim, É. (1912/2001) *The Elementary Forms of the Religious Life*. Oxford World Classics Edition. Oxford, UK and New York: Oxford University Press.

Elkins, D.N., Hedstrom, L.J., Hughes, L.L., Leaf, J.A. and Saunders, C. (1988) 'Toward a humanistic-phenomenological spirituality definition, description, and measurement.' *Journal of Humanistic Psychology 28*, 4, 5–18.

Engelhardt, H.T. (2003) 'The deChristianization of Christian hospital chaplaincy: Some bioethics reflections on professionalization, ecumenization, and secularization.' *Christian Bioethics 9*, 1, 139–160.

Fitzpatrick, J.J. and Whall, A.L. (1989) *Conceptual Models of Nursing: Analysis and Application* (second edition). Stamford, CT: Appleton and Lange.

Foster, J. (2007) 'Tribute to the theorists: Jean Watson over the years.' *Nursing Science Quarterly 20*, 1, 7.

Gallup (2012) *Gallup Daily Tracking*. Available at: www.gallup.com/poll/159785/rise-religious-nones-slows-2012.aspx, accessed 16 May 2015.

Handzo, G.F., Cobb, M., Holmes, C., Kelly, E. and Sinclair, S. (2014) 'Outcomes for professional health care chaplaincy: An international call to action.' *Journal of Healthcare Chaplaincy 20*, 2, 43–53.

Harrison, G. (2012) 'Exploring the relationship between the understanding of compassion and the practices of compassion in healthcare chaplaincy and other health care contexts.' *The Journal of Health Care Chaplaincy 12*, 2, 45–58.

Henderson, V. (1991) *The Nature of Nursing: A Definition of Its Implications for Practice, Research and Education – Reflections After 25 Years* (second revised edition). New York: National League for Nursing, USA.

Hinchliff, S.M., Norman, S.E. and Schober, J.E. (1989) *Nursing Practice and Health Care*. London: Edward Arnold.

Holloway, M. (2006) 'Death the great leveller? Towards a transcultural spirituality of dying and bereavement.' *Journal of Clinical Nursing 15*, 7, 833–839.

Hoogensen Gjorv, G. (2012) 'Security by any other name: Negative security, positive security, and a multi-actor security approach.' *Review of International Studies 38*, 835–859.

King, I.M. (1981) *A Theory of Nursing*. New York: Wiley.

Lachlan, G. (2008) 'Mindbody care: The ultimate patient experience?' *Scottish Journal of Healthcare Chaplaincy 11*, 2, 10–15.

Lane, K. (2006) 'The plasticity of professional boundaries: A case study of collaborative care in maternity services.' *Health Sociology Review 15*, 341–352.

LaRocca-Pitts, M. (2012) 'FACT, a chaplain's tool for assessing spiritual needs in an acute care setting.' *Chaplaincy Today 28*, 1, 25–32.

Lynch, G. (2012) *The Sacred and the Modern World: A Cultural Sociological Approach*. Oxford, UK: Oxford University Press.

McCarthy, M. (2000) 'Spirituality in a Postmodern Era.' In J. Woodward, S. Pattison and J. Patton (eds) *The Blackwell Reader in Pastoral and Practical Theology*. Malden, MA: Blackwell Publishers.

McGrath, P. (2003a) 'Religiosity and the challenge of terminal illness.' *Death Studies 27*, 10, 881–899.

McGrath, P. (2003b) 'Spiritual pain: A comparison of findings from survivors and hospice patients.' *American Journal of Hospice and Palliative Care 20*, 1, 23–33.

Mid Staffordshire NHS Foundation Trust, The (2013) 'Final report.' Available at: www.midstaffspublicinquiry.com/report (accessed 12 February 2015).

Moltmann, J. (1985) *God in Creation: An Ecological Doctrine of Creation*. Trans. Margaret Kohl. London: SCM.

Morris, D. (2003) 'Assisted suicide under the European Convention on Human Rights: A critique.' *European Human Rights Law Review 1*, 65–91.

Mowat, H. and Swinton, J. (2005) *What Do Chaplains Do? The Role of the Chaplain in Meeting the Spiritual Needs of Patients*. Aberdeen: Mowat Research Limited.

Naismith, S. (2001) 'Religion and the European Convention on Human Rights.' *Human Rights and UK Practice 2*, 1, 8.

National Secular Society (n.d.) 'Chaplaincy funding and the NHS.' Available at: www.secularism. org.uk/nhs-chaplaincy-funding.html (accessed 12 February 2015).

NHS (n.d.) 'NHS constitution.' Available at: www.nhs.uk/choiceintheNHS/Rightsand pledges/NHSConstitution/Pages/Overview.aspx (accessed 12 February 2015).

NHS Education Scotland (2008) 'Spiritual and religious care capabilities and competences for healthcare chaplains.' Available at: www.nes.scot.nhs.uk/education-and-training/ bydiscipline/spiritual-care/about-spiritual-care/publications.aspx (accessed 19 February 2015).

NHS Education Scotland/Scottish Executive Health Department (2002) Spiritual Care in NHS Scotland. NHS HDL (2002) 76. Available at: www.sehd.scot.nhs.uk/mels/hdl2002_76.pdf (accessed 16th May 2015).

NHS England (n.d.) 'Compassion in practice – our culture of compassionate care.' Available at: www.england.nhs.uk/nursingvision (accessed 12 February 2015).

NHS England (2013) 'Promoting equality and tackling health inequalities.' Paper NHSE121313. December 2013.

NHS England (2014) 'NHS chaplaincy guidelines: promoting excellence in spiritual care.' Draft as at July 2014.

NHS England (2015) *NHS Chaplaincy Guidelines 2015: Promoting Excellence in Pastoral, Spiritual & Religious Care.* Available at: www.england.nhs.uk/wp-content/uploads/2015/03/nhs-chaplaincy-guidelines-2015.pdf (accessed 16 May 2015).

NHS Scotland (2007) 'Standards for NHS Scotland chaplaincy services.' Available at: www.nes. scot.nhs.uk/education-and-training/by-discipline/spiritual-care/about-spiritual-care/ publications/standards-for-nhsscotland-chaplaincy-services.aspx (accessed 9 June 2015).

Nightingale, F. (1858) 'Nursing the Sick.' In R. Quain (ed.) *A Dictionary of Medicine* (ninth edition). New York: Appleton.

Nightingale, F. (1859/1969) *Notes on Nursing: What it is and What it is Not.* New York: Dover.

Nolan, R.D.S. (2008) 'Chaplaincy in the United Kingdom: Religious care or spiritual care?' *PlainViews: An E-Newsletter for Chaplains and Other Spiritual Care Providers.*

Orchard, H.C. (2001) *Spirituality in Health Care Contexts.* London: Jessica Kingsley Publishers.

Ovey C. and White, R. (2006) *Jacobs and White: The European Convention on Human Rights* (fourth edition). Oxford, UK: Oxford University Press.

Paley, J. (2008) 'Spirituality and secularization: Nursing and the sociology of religion.' *Journal of Clinical Nursing 17*, 2, 175–186.

Pattison, S. (2001) 'Dumbing Down the Spirit.' In H.C. Orchard (ed.) *Spirituality in Healthcare Contexts.* London: Jessica Kingsley Publishers.

Pattison, S. (forthcoming) 'Situating Chaplaincy in the United Kingdom: The Acceptable Face of 'Religion"?' In C. Swift, M. Cobb and A.J. Todd (eds) *Handbook of Chaplaincy Studies.* Farnham, UK: Ashgate.

Peterson, S.M. (2005) 'Beerheide v Suthers: A case study concerning religion in prisons in the USA.' *Ecclesiastical Law Journal 8*, 36, 67–73.

Pew Forum on Religion and Public Life (2008) 'U.S. religious landscape survey.' Washington, DC: Pew Research Center.

Pew Forum on Religion and Public Life (2012) 'U.S. religious landscape survey.' Washington, DC: Pew Research Center.

Puchalski, C. and Romer, A.L. (2000) 'Taking a spiritual history allows clinicians to understand patients more fully.' *Journal of Palliative Medicine 3*, 1, 129–137.

Reynolds, T.E. (2008) *Vulnerable Communion: A Theology of Disability and Hospitality.* Grand Rapids, MI: Brazos Press.

Rights, P. (2009) 'Encyclopedia of everyday law.' E-notes.com.

Rosenberg, A. (2006) 'Utilizing the language of Jean Watson's Caring Theory within a computerized clinical documentation system.' *CIN: Computers, Informatics, Nursing 24*, 1, 53–56.

Rozakis, C. (1998) *The Case-Law of the Commission as Regards Freedom of Thought, Conscience and Religion.* Baden-Baden, Germany:Nomos.

School of Environment and Development (n.d.) 'Multi-faith spaces – symptoms and agents of religious and social change.' SED, University of Manchester. Available at: www.sed. manchester.ac.uk/architecture/research/mfs/ (accessed 12 February 2015).

Scottish Executive Health Department HDL (2002) Spiritual Care in NHS Scotland.

Shelly, J.A. (2000) *Spiritual Care.* Downer's Grove, IL: Inter-Varsity Press.

Smith-Stoner, M. (2007) 'End-of-life preferences for atheists.' *Journal of Palliative Medicine 10,* 4, 923–928.

Snorton, T. (2006) 'Setting common standards for professonal chaplains in an age of diversity.' *Southern Medical Journal 99,* 6, 660–662.

South Yorkshire Workforce Development Confederation (2003) 'Caring for the spirit: A strategy for the chaplaincy and spiritual healthcare workforce.' London: South Yorkshire Workforce Development Confederation.

South Yorkshire Workforce Development Confederation (2004) 'Consultative proposals for a minimum data set for spiritual healthcare. Caring for the spirit: Implementation plan. Guidance Note 5.' London: South Yorkshire Workforce Development Confederation.

Speck, P. (2004) 'Spiritual care in health care.' *Scottish Journal of Healthcare Chaplaincy 7,* 1, 21–25.

Strang, S. and Strang, P. (2002) 'Questions posed to hospital chaplains by palliative care patients.' *Journal of Palliative Medicine 5,* 6, 857–864.

Sulmasy, D. (2006) *The Rebirth of the Clinic: An Introduction to Spirituality in Health Care.* Washington, DC: Georgetown University Press.

Swift, C. (2009) *Hospital Chaplaincy in the 21st Century: The Crisis of Spiritual Care on the NHS.* Aldershot, UK: Ashgate.

Swift, C. (2014) *Hospital Chaplaincy in the Twenty-first Century: The Crisis of Spiritual Care on the NHS* (second edition). Farnham/Burlington, VT: Ashgate.

Sword, D. (2009) 'Professionalization of conflict resolvers.' Mediate.com. Available at: www. mediate.com/articles/swordL7.cfm (accessed 19 February 2015).

Taylor, C. (2004) *Modern Social Imaginaries.* Durham, NC and London: Duke University Press.

Telegraph, The (2009) 'Chaplains costing NHS £32 million a year.' *The Telegraph,* 9 April. Available at: www.telegraph.co.uk/news/religion/5123378/Chaplains-costing-NHS-32-million-a-year.html (accessed 19 February 2015).

Todd, A.J. (2011) 'Responding to Diversity: Chaplaincy in a Multi-Faith Context.' In M. Threlfall-Holmes and M. Newitt (eds) *Being a Chaplain.* London: SPCK.

Todd, A.J. (2013) 'Preventing the "neutral" chaplain? The potential impact of anti-"extremism" policy on prison chaplaincy.' *Practical Theology 6,* 2, 144–158.

Todd, A.J. (2014) 'Religion, security, rights, the individual and rates of exchange: Religion in negotiation with British public policy in prisons and the military.' *International Journal of Politics, Culture and Society* (online).

Todd, A.J. and Tipton, L. (2011) 'The role and contribution of a multi-faith prison chaplaincy to the contemporary prison service, research report to the National Offender Management Service.' Available at: http://stmichaels.ac.uk/chaplaincy-studies/centre-reports-and-publications (accessed 19 February 2015).

Tournier, P. (1986) *A Listening Ear: Fifty Years as a Doctor of the Whole Person. Texts Selected by Charles Piquet.* London: Hodder and Stoughton.

Underwood, L.G. and Teresi, J.A. (2002) 'The daily spiritual experience scale: Development, theoretical description, reliability, exploratory factor analysis, and preliminary construct validity using health-related data.' *Annals of Behavioral Medicine 24,* 1, 22–33.

UK Board of Healthcare Chaplaincy (2009) 'Spiritual and religious care capabilities and competences for healthcare chaplains.' Available at: www.ukbhc.org.uk (accessed 31 October 2014).

Unruh, A.M., Versnel, J. and Kerr, N. (2002) 'Spirituality unplugged: A review of commonalities and contentions, and a resolution.' *Canadian Journal of Occupational Therapy. Revue Canadienne D'ergothérapie 69,* 1, 5–19.

Vasquez, M.A. and Marquardt, M.F. (2003) *Globalizing the Sacred: Religion Across the Americas.* Piscataway, NJ: Rutgers University Press; London: Eurospan.

Viktor Frankl Institut (2014) 'What is logotherapy and existential analysis?' Available at: www.viktorfrankl.org/e/logotherapy.html (accessed 19 February 2015).

Viktor Frankl Institute of Logotherapy (2014) 'Logotherapy.' Available at: www.logotherapyinstitute.org/About_Logotherapy.html (accessed 19 February 2015).

Watson, J. (ed.) (1994) *Applying the Art and Science of Human Caring.* New York: NLN Publications.

Watson, J. (2005) *Caring Science as Sacred Science.* Philadelphia, PA: F.A. Davis.

Watson, J. (2008) *Nursing: The Philosophy and Science of Caring* (revised edition). Boulder, CO: University Press of Colorado.

Welford, L. (2011) 'Spiritual healthcare and public policy: An investigation into the legal and social policy frameworks of healthcare chaplaincy.' Unpublished PhD thesis, Cardiff University.

Welsh Assembly Government (2010) 'Standards for spiritual care services in the NHS in Wales. Available at: http://gov.wales/docs/dhss/publications/100525spiritualcarestandardsen.pdf (accessed 9 June 2015).

Wohlrab-Sahra, M. and Burchardt, M. (2012) 'Multiple secularities: Toward a cultural sociology of secular modernities.' *Comparative Sociology 11,* 875–909.

Woodhead, L. and Heelas, P. (2000) *Religion in Modern Times, an Interpretive Anthology.* Malden, MA: Blackwell Publishing.

World Health Organization (1946) WHO *definition of Health.* Available at: www.who.int/about/definition/en/print.html (accessed 10 June 2015).

YouGov (n.d.) 'Archive.' Available at: http://yougov.co.uk/publicopinion/archive/?category=politics&sort=-label&page=2 (accessed 12 February 2015).

Other sources (Welford)

Letter dated 10 March 2004, written from the British Humanist Association to the Secretary of State for Health. This is available on the British Humanist Association's website, at: www.humanism.org.uk/site/cms/contentviewarticle.asp?article=1643andsplash=yes (accessed 19 February 2015).

Article on the National Secular Society's website, which supports the cutting of hospital chaplains' posts within NHS Trusts: www.secularism.org.uk/atlasthospitalchaplainsintheline.html (accessed 19 February 2015).

PART 3

Researching Spiritual Care

CHAPTER 9

Making Spiritual Care Visible

The Developing Agenda and Methodologies
for Research in Spiritual Care

Steve Nolan

Introduction

Since 1990 the growth in articles published about spirituality and
healthcare has been 'exponential' (Mowat 2008, p.24). A search of the
term 'spiritual care' on NHS Library databases (AMED, BNI, CINAHL,
EMBASE, Health Business Elite, HMIC, Medline, PsycINFO) yields 42
results for the year 1990–1991, rising to 440 for the year 2012–2013.
Significantly, this increase has been driven, not by those for whom
spiritual care is their specialty, namely chaplains, but by a variety of
healthcare professionals interested in and concerned about spiritual
care. As a consequence, the field of spiritual care has been developed
by non-specialists, mainly nurses. This observation implies no criticism
of healthcare professional colleagues; but the situation is anomalous: in
which other healthcare field have the parameters been determined by
non-specialists? There is no argument that spiritual care is an integral
part of a nurse's role (Goodhead 2008). The problem is not with nurses,
but with the knowledge vacuum they and others have felt obliged to fill.

There are signs that the situation is changing, albeit slowly. Yet
the lack of spiritual care specialists actively engaging in spiritual care
research represents an important deficit, precisely because contemporary
healthcare is missing the specialist knowledge and experience that
chaplains have to offer.

In this chapter, I will review developments within chaplaincy
research. Focusing first on the emerging imperative for chaplaincy to

demonstrate its efficacy, the chapter contrasts evidence-based practice with practice-based evidence. After detailing several examples of practice-based evidence, the chapter introduces the research of three serving healthcare chaplains.

Evidence-based practice: The emerging imperative in spiritual care research

Writing his second editorial for the *Scottish Journal of Healthcare Chaplaincy* in 1999, John Swinton characterised a situation in which research- and evidence-based practice had little 'immediate impact on the day to day practice' of many Scottish chaplains (Swinton 1999, p.1). What was true for Scottish chaplains was true for their southern colleagues. In part, this was because the concept of evidence-based practice, described as 'the conscientious, explicit, and judicious use of current best evidence in making decisions about the care of individual patients' (Sackett *et al.* 1996), was a relatively new and still somewhat contested idea within the NHS (Carr-Hill 1995). For this reason, Swinton included a paper by Vanora Hundley (1999), a lecturer and researcher in nursing studies, which introduced and explained the concept as it relates to chaplaincy.

Awareness of the impact of research was perhaps more advanced in the practice of US chaplains; probably because the economics of North American healthcare had already exposed those chaplains to the vicissitudes of market forces. Even so, the US picture was mixed. Writing in the same edition of the *Scottish Journal of Healthcare Chaplaincy* as Hundley, Noel Brown (1999) cited Larry VandeCreek and George Fitchett as examples of US chaplains 'working to establish new paradigms for chaplaincy', in contrast to those who 'continue to function as they did half a century ago' (Brown 1999, p.16). The crisis Brown identified had already been made explicit in the first edition of the US *Journal of Health Care Chaplaincy*, in which Elisabeth McSherry, a medical doctor, warned that chaplaincy departments needed to modernise their discipline by utilising 'objective instruments for clinical care and for management reporting', and that this was necessary, 'not only for quality of patient care but also for longterm [*sic*] survival of chaplain departments' (McSherry 1987, p.3).

Almost 30 years on, the imperative of McSherry's advice remains pertinent on both sides of the Atlantic, particularly as healthcare providers are pressed to reduce operational costs. The experience of

Worcester Acute Hospitals NHS Trust, in 2006, is but the most high-profile case of a British Trust's decision to cut chaplaincy provision on the basis of a need to improve financial performance (Swift 2009, pp.81–95). While the heat of this particular crisis may have dissipated, the place of spiritual care within healthcare continues to be scrutinised and its provision from public funds questioned by those with a secularist agenda (Christian 2011).

Concern with the survival of the profession is, however, a defensive reason for engaging in research. More positive is the desire to improve the delivery of spiritual care. In 2003, the South Yorkshire Workforce Development Confederation (WDC) published 'Caring for the spirit', a modernising strategy aiming at enabling the spiritual healthcare workforce to 'match the changes in healthcare and in spirituality within the UK' (South Yorkshire Workforce Development Confederation 2003, p.5). The strategy gives research- and evidence-based practice strong support (South Yorkshire Workforce Development Confederation 2003, p.18), proposing that all chaplains should have access to research training and acknowledging that, while only a small number of chaplains (around 1–2%) will be 'research active', all chaplains should be 'research aware' (South Yorkshire Workforce Development Confederation 2003, p.19) – a distinction that is now widely recognised (Cobb 2008; Fitchett and Grossoehme 2012; Speck 2005). Importantly, 'Caring for the spirit' identifies the need to uncover 'the evidence which supports efficacy in spiritual healthcare' (South Yorkshire Workforce Development Confederation 2003, p.20). Two notable initiatives followed: a standard for research was developed (www. ukbhc.org.uk/research/research-information; see Speck 2005); and NHS UK) commissioned a review of the research literature to identify and grade 'the published evidence about structure, role and efficacy of healthcare chaplaincy' (South Yorkshire Workforce Development Confederation 2003, p.20).

Harriet Mowat's (2008) review of 142 articles published since 1990 found that the research literature 'as it stands does not directly or substantially address the issue of efficacy in healthcare chaplaincy' (Mowat 2008, p.31; see Fitchett and Grossoehme 2012 for a similar evaluation of the state of US chaplaincy research). However, Mowat identifies and analyses eight categories of issues that she argues represent the focus of concern within UK healthcare chaplaincy: definitions of spirituality and religion; the relationship between spirituality and well-being; understanding what would count as 'evidence' and 'efficacy';

the professionalisation of healthcare chaplaincy; who should deliver spiritual care; assessing spiritual need; patient perspectives; and multi-faith issues (Mowat 2008, p.32). Perhaps most usefully, Mowat sets 'the current profile of chaplaincy research against the patient's journey in healthcare settings' (Mowat 2008, p.7). The value of this is in identifying existing and potential areas for chaplaincy research as they relate to that journey: an evidence base to show *what happens* and that *what happens is valuable* in terms of intended outcomes and enhanced well-being (Mowat 2008, pp.71, 72). From this, Mowat concludes that one of the most important tasks for healthcare chaplaincy research is to investigate the outputs of the care chaplains deliver (Mowat 2008, p.74), and she lists potential areas for research correlated against the stages of the patients' journey through the healthcare services, including screening and assessment, treatment and care planning, and improvement of health and well-being (Mowat 2008, pp.75–77).

South Yorkshire Workforce Development Confederation's vision of modernising the research aspect of spiritual healthcare by 2010 may have been overly optimistic. Notwithstanding the fact that Mowat's review has been followed by an encouraging increase in chaplaincy-related research, Swinton's characterisation of chaplaincy remains relevant. This is because, as Mark Cobb observes, healthcare chaplains:

> *are predominantly formed by theological education, pastoral care training and the humanities, which may have some underpinnings in research-related subjects including biblical studies, history, ecclesiology, psychology and sociology. However, most chaplains are not trained in research methods and, while they may practise forms of theological reflection, few apply recognized methods of critical inquiry and analysis. (Cobb 2008, p.5)*

The disconnect is that evidence-based research is *empirical* research and on the whole chaplains lack the relevant training and experience to provide the empirical evidence to address Swinton's question: 'How can one "prove" that chaplaincy "works?"' (Swinton 1999, 1).

Swinton's question is salient, although epistemologically it poses its own questions about the nature of scientific knowledge: how we know what we know, and on what basis we claim our knowledge as scientific. These questions go beyond the scope of this chapter, yet they regularly find expression when chaplains claim 'We know that chaplaincy "works" because we see in our daily experience that people respond to our care; they tell us that they find benefit in what we do for them, so why would we *want* to try to "prove" what we already know?' In response, the argument is that evidence-based practice, with its associated 'gold-standard' technique, the randomised controlled trial/randomised clinical trial (RCT), has been responsible for changing healthcare for the better, effecting a shift in healthcare culture and 'increasing the *accountability* and *transparency* of healthcare decision making' (Bower and Gilbody 2010, p.17). This is because, while evidence-based practice acknowledges a range of evidence types, 'from the most rigorous scientific research, through less rigorous forms of research, personal clinical experience and the opinions of experts', it also imposes a hierarchy on the trustworthiness of evidence, in which 'higher forms…trump lower forms' (Bower and Gilbody 2010, p.5). In this case, the assertion 'chaplaincy works' may count as a form of expert opinion, but only as a lower form of evidence.

The association of evidence-based practice with RCTs has become so strong that there is a common tendency to assume that 'evidence' is always and only ever quantitative (Fitchett 2011, p.4; Hundley 1999, p.12); in other words, that qualitative evidence is of little to no value. However, the limitations of RCTs have been argued, particularly in terms of the capacity of RCTs to demonstrate the efficacy of psychological therapies (Wampold 2010, p.xvii) – which involve interventions whose qualities are arguably related to those of spiritual care – and in terms of their relevance to the current needs of chaplaincy studies (Fitchett 2011, p.4). From the perspective of psychological therapies, 'practice-based evidence', which measures the progress of patients across the course of therapy (Wampold 2010, p.xviii), offers one possible approach to answering Swinton's question about efficacy. Not as a way of providing evidence to replace RCTs, but as a way of providing evidence that complements and completes RCTs (Barkham *et al.* 2010; Nolan 2011), and as a way of providing 'the evidence most vital to the patient sitting in the consulting room' (Wampold 2010, p.xviii) – or the person in the hospital bed.

Practice-based evidence

As Handzo *et al.* (2014) note, practice-based evidence is 'a much needed first-step for chaplaincy' because it 'values chaplains' tacit knowledge and grows the evidence base from the ground up' (Handzo *et al.* 2014, p.49). At a most basic level, service evaluations or audits provide data for evidence that is practice-based. However, the development of tools that can measure the outcomes of chaplains' spiritual care interventions offer the potential for gathering data that are directly relevant to the task of demonstrating the efficacy of both chaplaincy and spiritual care. For example, all chaplains know from experience the benefit their empathic listening has for people who need to talk. Such knowledge from experience would not qualify as a high-level form of evidence; however, the *experience of those who have benefited from being listened to*, when reported and captured, represents the kind of outcome data that can be utilised as a form of practice-based evidence.

Patient Reported Outcome Measure

The so-called 'Lothian PROM' is the first Patient Reported Outcome Measure (PROM) to have been developed as a way of measuring spiritual care (Snowden *et al.* 2013a). Developed from a review of the literature (with particular reference to Mowat and Swinton's (2007) report, 'What do chaplains do?'), the Lothian PROM has been validated by two groups of experienced chaplains attending professional conferences (2011 and 2012) and tested with a patient population (Snowden *et al.* 2013b).

The Lothian PROM invites patients to respond to a short questionnaire, divided into five sections. Section One concerns basic demographic information: age, gender and length of hospital stay. Sections Two through Four invite participants to use a five-point Likert-scale (ranging from 'not at all' to 'all the time') to respond to a number of statements grouped under three headings: (§2) 'During my meeting with the chaplain I felt…'; (§3) 'After meeting with the chaplain'; (§4) 'Statements that describe me now'. The final section (§5) provides a free text box in which participants can respond to the invitation: 'Please add any final comments you wish to make about how the chaplain's input affected you' (Snowden *et al.* 2013a). For the purpose of statistical analysis, the Likert-scale responses are assigned numerical values (rank) – 1 representing 'not at all'; 5 representing 'all the time' – and analysed statistically using the 'Spearman's rho' formula to expose correlations between responses. Of particular interest are the correlations uncovered between §2 and §3, which demonstrate a particularly clear correlation between people reporting 'I was able to talk about what was on my mind' (a statement in §2) and all the measured outcomes of §3 ('I could be honest with myself about how I was really feeling'; 'My levels of anxiety had lessened'; 'I had gained a better perspective on my illness/

the illness of my relative/friend'; 'Things seemed under control again'; 'A sense of peace I had not felt before') (Snowden *et al.* 2013b, p.19).

From these data, Snowden *et al.* infer that 'the activity of creating the conditions to allow people to speak freely' has 'clear empirical benefit' (Snowden *et al.* 2013b, p.20). This inference may seem unremarkable, but the point is that it is based on outcomes as reported by patients. As such, this empirical evidence derived from practice can become the basis for further research and, for example,

> *studies could be designed to test the prediction that being able to talk about what is currently important would lessen anxiety and give a sense of control and peace. If this study could establish that being able to talk about what is currently important causes a lowering of anxiety then this would value the skills of chaplains (and others) in facilitating the conditions for allowing people to talk as an end in itself. (Snowden et al. 2013b, p.19)*

User-centred research

Patient-reported outcomes are a version of user-centred research. Foskett (2013) describes an important user-centred research project in which he participated as both 'a user of mental health services and a spiritual and religious adviser to a Mental Health Foundation Trust' (Foskett 2013, p.86). Using patients as the subjects of research opens important ethical concerns, which rightly need to be addressed to the satisfaction of the appropriate Research Ethics Committee (www.nres.nhs.uk). However, there is good evidence that patients or service users want to participate in research (Terry *et al.* 2006), either out of an altruistic motivation or to improve their own future care (Bevan *et al.* 1993).

The research group Foskett describes included 'users/survivors of the mental health services in Somerset' (Nicholls 2002, p.6), all with personal experience of mental ill-health, spirituality and religion. The group identified questions important to service users/survivors whose spirituality and/or religion were important. The questions were piloted in order to focus the research around the experience of mental health and religious/spiritual needs in relation to help/hindrance experienced from mental health services and/or local religious and spiritual groups. Over a period of six months (2000–2001) the research group interviewed a mixed group of Christians, pagans and those with 'non-religious spiritualities', all of whom 'were or had been in contact with mental health services in Somerset and who were interested in...spirituality and/or religion' (Nicholls 2002, p.7). The findings, reported in 'Taken seriously: The Somerset spirituality project' (Nicholls 2002), expose the reality that 'service users had more confidence in their religious and spiritual beliefs, and how they affected their mental health, than did either the mental health professionals or the clergy' (Foskett 2013, p.88).

While such user-centred research projects may not directly address Swinton's question about the efficacy of chaplaincy, they nonetheless highlight the perceived importance many people attach to the place and value of spirituality and religion in their healthcare. Significantly, they also model an approach to research methodology that is more or less explicitly critical of the evidence-based approach, and offers an approach that runs counter to the dominant research culture. As a modernist research methodology (Denzin and Lincoln 2000, p.14), evidence-based research is predicated on a set of realist assumptions about ontology (the nature of reality) and epistemology (the nature and status of knowledge). In brief, realist ontology assumes that reality (the everyday world) is objective and external, and that consequently unbiased data can be collected and verified by carefully following technical procedures (Charmaz 2000, p.510).

As researchers who were also users of mental health services, the Somerset Spirituality Project researchers admit to their 'strong personal interest in the subject' (Nicholls 2002, p.6). In so doing, they acknowledge that they are epistemologically implicated in their research. Their interpretation of the data is not objective and unbiased, nor is it intended to be. Rather, they acknowledge it as a 'construction' that is, by definition, contaminated by the researchers' values and perspectives, which they endeavour to make explicit (in a way that modernist research methodologies are only expected to do in relation to vested financial interest). A further important distinction of user-centred research projects is a concern with empowering users. Again, this is in contrast to the dominant research model, which by its objectification serves to disempower its subjects. As Foskett puts it, 'The transformation from doing to, to being with, is not easily absorbed by a service in which assessment and delivery are so central' (Foskett 2013, p.85). User-centred research regards users as collaborators in a cooperative enquiry.

Action research

User-centred research is less a research methodology than a research philosophy that regards participants as collaborators in a cooperative enquiry. Action research is typically a form of collaborative enquiry that uses a community of practice to address specific issues or solve a given problem. Mowat, Bunniss and Kelly (2012) describe the Community Chaplaincy Listening (CCL) project, which employs an action research method to address the challenge faced by healthcare professionals, who are required to listen to patients but not given sufficient time to do so. In this project, chaplains are actively involved in gathering and reflecting on data as researchers and practitioners, within 'a framework for practice…[which] provides continuous feedback to the participants so that changes and developments can be negotiated based on evidence' (Mowat *et al.* 2012, p.22).

Begun in 2010, and currently in its third stage, CCL is an ongoing national programme, instigated by the Healthcare Chaplaincy Training and Development Unit of NHS Education for Scotland and supported by the Scottish Government. The first stage invited four chaplains to co-create with researchers a 'spiritual listening intervention' to be based in GP surgeries. Patients referred for the intervention met with the chaplaincy listener and were invited to 'tell their story' with a view to considering 'the existential issues they are facing' and finding 'some sense of resolution or peace with what is currently happening in their life'. They were offered as many 50-minute sessions as they needed and were free 'to discharge themselves from the listening service at any time, without explanation' (Mowat *et al.* 2012, pp.21–22). The action research method was used to guide data collection (from patients, GPs, chaplains and managers, via questionnaires and semi-structured interviews) and assess the findings (patients found CCL overwhelmingly positive; GPs found CCL helpful; chaplains found CCL largely positive; and managers reported they would like to see CCL as part of a suite of talking therapies) (Mowat *et al.* 2012, p.23).

An important distinctive of action research is that findings inform further rounds of action. From this first stage, the researchers found they needed to clarify both the purpose and the process of CCL. These learning points informed the second stage of the study, which subsequently found the purpose of the service had become clearer, at least to some.

Those using the service reported that 'the predominant activity was that they talked and the chaplain listened'; they felt they were able to 'speak freely about whatever they wanted to'; that they 'had the sense that the Chaplain was giving them his/her undivided attention'; that they 'felt able to tell the whole story from beginning to end without being interrupted'; that 'the chaplain was non-judgemental, did not attempt to label them and remained right with them throughout the experience'; and that the 'issue of the service being spiritual listening delivered by a chaplain did not appear to be a barrier' (Bunniss, Mowat and Snowden 2013, p.47). For their part, the chaplains' descriptions were:

> *highly resonant with the patients' descriptions of what happens in a CCL session. They confirmed that the main activity was to listen, hold, reflect back and sum up the patient story. They saw themselves as providing a safe, accepting space and a sincere relationship by which the patient could feel able to tell their story. (Bunniss et al. 2013, p.49)*

In contrast, GPs reported that they remained 'unsure about how best to describe the service to patients' (Bunniss *et al.* 2013, p.48), with some feeling 'nervous' using the terms 'chaplain' or 'spiritual'. With regard to the need to clarify the process of CCL, the GPs continued to express their wish for 'more feedback and communication with the chaplains', with many saying they had 'no real engagement with the chaplain' (Bunniss *et al.* 2013, p.49).

> *In terms of addressing how to prove that chaplaincy 'works' (Swinton 1999, p.1), the value of action research like this is obvious. Action research also has value in terms of service development. The inherent action-reflection model on which the methodology depends will be familiar to many who have been trained in practical theology, and for this reason action research 'is used increasingly in practical theological empirical research. (Mowat et al. 2012, p.22).*

Empirical theology

As a relevant aside, it is worth highlighting here the theological sub-discipline of empirical theology. Emerging in the 1980s in the work of Johannes van der Ven (1998), empirical theology is essentially concerned with finding 'the divine or the holy within the relations that gather up the fragments of the world' (Corrington 1998, p.166). To this end, Van der Ven proposed that theologians should adopt the perspectives, tools and methodologies of the social sciences. Leslie Francis extends this to include the idea that empirical theologians should allow their work to be scrutinised, 'not only by other theologians, but also by other social scientists working outside the theological academy' (Francis, Robbins and Astley 2009, p.xiv). For Francis and other British empirical theologians, 'empirical theology is concerned with those kinds of theological data that are properly amenable to empirical investigation' (Francis *et al.* 2009, p.xiii), and they suggest, for example, that empirical investigation can illuminate 'questions about the nature of God and about the nature of humankind...especially in light of the assertion that both women and men are created in the divine image' (Francis *et al.* 2009, p.xiv). The sub-discipline is supported by the International Society of Empirical Research in Theology, the *Journal of Empirical Theology* and book series published by Ashgate (Explorations in Practical, Pastoral and Empirical Theology) and Brill (Empirical Studies in Theology).

Case study

Although not considered 'research' in the strictest sense, and certainly not in the sense understood by NHS research ethics committees, case studies of chaplaincy and spiritual care interventions are an important way of investigating how chaplaincy works. In fact, unlike the psychotherapeutic disciples that are closely related to spiritual care, case studies have been significantly under-developed by chaplaincy. US chaplain, George Fitchett, has argued that case studies are vital for 'developing the foundation from which more advanced studies can be developed' (Fitchett 2011, pp.4–5). His point is that before chaplains – or, for that matter, any healthcare professional – can begin to study the efficacy of a spiritual care intervention, accurate and detailed descriptions of spiritual care are needed.

Fitchett details a three-stage model of research, drawn from research in behavioural therapies. The first stage, which focuses on the basic elements of the therapeutic intervention and how to measure its effects, has two parts: Stage 1A develops a detailed description, or protocol, of the intervention. The protocol demonstrates, with case examples, the feasibility of the intervention and selects appropriate measures to test its effects. Stage 1B pilots the intervention, again in a small number of cases, looking for evidence of the intended effects and for any associated negative effects. Only when this work is complete do investigators move to Stage 2, testing the intervention's efficacy in an RCT. Finally,

Stage 3 examines the intervention in clinical practice. Fitchett argues that, before chaplains do Stage 2 research, chaplains need to lay the foundations of Stage 1A and 1B.

> *This is where case studies come in. We need good case studies to provide detailed information about three things that are part of Stage 1A research: 1) descriptions of the patient (or family) to whom we provided care, 2) descriptions of the spiritual care that was provided, and 3) descriptions of the changes that occurred as a result of that spiritual care. (Fitchett 2011, p.5)*

Regrettably, Fitchett has found almost no case studies that provide the kind of detail he argues is needed.

Since 2011, Fitchett has been pioneering a project to encourage chaplains to publish case studies. Fitchett's project has led to three published cases (Cooper 2011; King 2012; Risk 2013 – each accompanied by critique/comment from a chaplain and a healthcare professional from a related discipline) and a book-length collection of nine cases (Fitchett and Nolan 2015). While case studies do not require approval from a research ethics committee, they nevertheless present their own set of ethical difficulties, particularly around confidentiality and permission to publish. For example, protecting patient confidentiality is essential, disguising the case material will probably impact on the descriptive quality of the case, which in turn have implications on its value for further research. These ethical issues are considered by McCurdy and Fitchett (2011).

Recent research by serving healthcare chaplains

The chapters that follow represent recent postgraduate work undertaken by chaplains working in the Cardiff Centre for Chaplaincy Studies. Mental health chaplain Julian Raffay reports on work he has published elsewhere (2012, 2013) on developing a spiritual assessment tool for use in mental health. His chapter includes something of his personal experience as a chaplain researcher/practitioner. Working in the Acute sector, Karen MacKinnon describes an important study, a mixed-method, cross-sectional survey addressing the question of the secularity of the NHS, with particular reference to the beliefs and values of volunteers. As well as contributing to chaplaincy studies, these chapters are encouraging examples of what can be achieved by chaplain researcher/practitioners.

CHAPTER 10

Researching Spiritual Care in a Mental Health Context

Julian Raffay

Introduction

In this chapter I describe something of the experience of researching spiritual care in the context of a Master's dissertation. I aim to provide insights that will be helpful for anyone considering or interested in similar research. I explore my experience of developing a research proposal, consider the research process, look at issues involved in administering the research and then conclude with reflections on the impact of the research.

Like many research topics spiritual care has both conceptual and clinical aspects to it. It does not lend itself easily to definition, yet is recognised as significant in terms of an individual service user's desire for quality of service provision. It is also, inevitably, a political matter as it competes for both finite resources and the attention of over-busy staff.

In this chapter I would like to add to the work of Faulkner (2012), who first drew my attention to the matter of user empowerment within the research process itself. Though current governance frameworks work against it, and ethics committees seem strangely blind to the injustice of doing research *to* rather than *with* the participants, I am convinced that a radically different approach is not only long overdue but will also lead to richer findings. My hope is that, in mental health research at least, service users will be given every opportunity to decide what matters warrant researching and to work in collaboration with skilled researchers in shaping projects at every stage, right through to dissemination. I further hope that service users or survivors, some of whom are competent researchers themselves, will have their work recognised as being of at least equal worth. Anything else risks either patronising or further disempowering this group of people, whose legitimate right to describe their own experiences and make meaningful choices has often been taken away by powerful others. Arguably, this continues to be the case.

As I look back on my own work, I do so with regret that I did not have the imagination or courage at the time to appreciate that my work could, theoretically at least, have involved rather than consulted service users through the entire research cycle. In fairness, the thinking behind documents such as 'Good practice guidance for involving people with experience of mental health problems in research' (NIHR 2013) was in its early stages when I started out, though co-production in other fields has been common practice for many years (e.g. Lassiter 2005).

Developing the research proposal

I was convinced that the subject of my research needed to emerge from my context as a mental health chaplain. I asked myself three broad questions: (i) what issues needed to be addressed; (ii) what was going on in the literature; and (iii) what skills could I bring to bear? In terms of the issues to be addressed, I reflected on different aspects of what was going on around me and considered what I was struggling with. I found that the hardest part of my job was training nurses and support workers in spirituality. They quite simply did not get it. They found the language and thought forms inaccessible, and they struggled to see its relevance to their day-to-day work with service users. I felt as if I was perhaps on to something, but needed to check out the literature in order to verify whether my frustrations reflected a more widespread problem. Though hardly a literature review, an initial database search and a few emails to researchers and friends confirmed that I was not the only one with this experience.

Encouraged by the thought that I had found something worth exploring, I asked myself what skills I might have to bring into the situation. I considered what skills I already had and what I might be able to acquire. I realised that my psychology background provided me with the tools to produce a questionnaire. I was also confident that I could learn the research skills required to conduct interviews and extract meaningful data from them. It felt as if I had found my prospective research area, which involved the use of Grounded Theory to explore the perceptions of mental health service users and nurses around spirituality and spiritual care.

The supervisor

In choosing a supervisor, I found it helpful to give some thought as to what I might need to help me to complete the research process, and specifically where my personal weaknesses lay. At a very practical level, I forgot to budget for travel costs to meet my supervisor and had to find more money than I had allowed for.

My supervisor was remarkably supportive and could not have done more to help, but there were times when I felt exasperated by the detailed revisions that he entirely appropriately suggested. At times I felt dispirited, but I also discovered that persistence and accepting responsibility for the progress of my work were essential prerequisites for success.

The research question

One of the first tasks my supervisor did was to help me to turn my early ideas into a carefully worded research question. A good research question will be concise and intelligible. It needed to demonstrate that I had thought clearly about what I was hoping to find and how I intended to go about it. It marks the 'destination' of the research and, as I found myself sucked into the detail at various stages, it served as a reference point against which I could periodically check to ensure that I was not heading off course. I refined it as I went along, but spent perhaps the best part of a fortnight working on it and found that the effort up front more than paid off.

My own research title covered much of the ground but failed to indicate the methodology: 'What are the factors that prevent or enable the development of a spiritual assessment tool in mental health and that stand in the way of or facilitate the provision of quality spiritual care?'

The relationship between methodology and findings

In just the same way that a worker will pick the appropriate tool from their tool kit, I needed to choose the appropriate research methodology to achieve my intended purpose. Yet I also needed to recognise that my choice of tool would influence what I might discover. This impact may be far from easy to identify. I considered Action Research as a methodology, and was drawn to its focus on bringing about meaningful change in the system or organisation for the benefit of a socially disadvantaged group, but felt that the same values could be applied to other methodologies in order to bring about similar outcomes. I chose Constructivist Grounded Theory because it recognises the researcher as part of the findings. It recognises that, as a chaplain, I am likely to find certain things, whereas a nurse researcher might find others. Equally, because participants know me to be a chaplain, they might choose to talk to me about different matters than had I been a member of their ward nursing team. I specifically chose Charmaz's (2006) particular methodology because I found it clear and workable.

Objectivist and constructivist perspectives

Coming to grips with the philosophical poles of objectivism and constructivism is but one additional challenge of Grounded Theory and similar research. While objectivists seek to control for and eliminate investigator effects, constructivists work with them, seeing their findings as being jointly shaped by themselves as investigators and by the participants. I was strongly aware that the very idea of my research emerged from my involvement in it, yet seemed to require a new perspective. I faced the challenge of taking on a new and temporary role as researcher, only later to revert to my day-to-day role as chaplain. This difficult task was not simply going to be addressed by wearing an ordinary shirt as opposed to a clerical collar. I dealt with it in part by promising participants that I would never mention the research subsequently unless they first brought the matter up. In that regard, at least, I was successful!

The research proposal

If the research question is the destination, then the research proposal is the map. The proposal spells out in considerable detail how the research will be conducted. It is an important part of the research process and helps to crystallise thinking. Just as a building's intended purpose will influence its design, so too the purpose of the research should shape the design of a research proposal. I recognise now that the validity of my research would have been all the greater, and I would have found it much easier to get service users and carers to participate, had I more fully involved them in the entire research process. One option might have been to have recruited service user/carer research consultants from one ward or unit and participants from another. Had I involved service users and carers throughout, the whole endeavour would also have been far more enriching, even if at times harder to manage with the extra meetings that would have had to be scheduled. There would also have been the matter of fair remuneration.

When I sought to write my research proposal, I was uncertain as to what was expected. I simply Googled the phrase 'grounded theory research proposal', identified which elements of the search results suited my purpose and then put mine together. I showed this to a small number of service users and carers, and checked it out with a number of people who had written their own.

The research timetable

I found I needed at the very least a basic chart with target dates and deadlines, a kind of milometer to check that I was making sufficient progress towards the final write-up. At times, I was able to get ahead. At other times, I found myself waiting for clearance, and so worked instead on something that was perhaps less urgent. I found a management technique called critical path analysis helpful in identifying the steps in the process that held everything up and ensured that I gave these the greatest attention. The technique requires two elements to be considered: things that take a long time (e.g. interviewing mental health service users) and activities that have to wait for the completion of other activities (in the jargon, dependencies, for example, waiting for research ethics approval before starting interviews). My approach was to start by drawing a diagram with arrows that illustrated what activity was dependent upon another. The second stage was to work out the timing for each part of the process. The critical path is the one that is likely to slow the whole operation down. A simpler approach is the Gantt chart (which does much the same thing by using bars to represent events in time), but this is not so good at allowing for unexpected delays. I found many illustrations of these approaches on the web.

Participants

I found myself having to think carefully about inclusion and exclusion criteria as part of the research proposal. Though it was far from my first choice, I took the decision only to include adults who were fluent in spoken English. With this exception, participants were expected to be reflective of the intended population (purposive sampling) from which they were drawn. Had I not done this, I might have ended up with only religious service users or staff, and it would have been harder to generalise my findings. In spite of seeking to cover the bases, decisions inevitably have to be taken around the unexpected. For instance, in spite of the fact that I had explicitly asked for trained staff (and service users), a couple of support workers signed up. I took the decision to interview them. They contributed rich and relevant data that I decided to keep in the study, as it was clear that no one would be harmed by these actions and I was explicit about their involvement.

Capacity to consent

When I started out, I had little idea how complex consent might be. I had imagined that it was nothing more than a matter of asking a participant to tick a box on a questionnaire. Far from it! For a start, the questionnaire had to be carefully worded to ensure that precisely what was being consented to was made explicit.

Second, informed consent requires capacity to consent. Capacity is defined in the Mental Capacity Act (HMSO 2005), which lays down five specific criteria for assessing capacity. I discovered that I had to understand what these criteria meant and adhere to them in the course of my recruitment and interviews.

Third, a person needs to be provided with opportunities to withdraw consent. However, because of the increasing consequences of such action for the researcher as the research progresses, the extent of their rights to do so will typically be diminished over time. In practice, a clause that states the participant may withdraw at any point up to the start of analysis might have provided a simple and balanced workaround. I experienced a couple of withdrawals of consent prior to interview, but had factored this into my research proposal by planning to recruit a few more participants than I anticipated needing.

In acute mental health settings, another aspect of capacity to consent is the matter of fluctuating capacity. Had I excluded participants with possibly fluctuating capacity *a priori*, I would have automatically excluded the experiences of a significant proportion of the acute psychiatric ward population. However, insofar as these people are deemed vulnerable adults, coercion becomes a real risk. I made every effort to avoid coercion, and arguably left myself without any ability to encourage service users to participate other than in response to my posters.

Sample size

A couple of concepts in Grounded Theory proved particularly helpful in obtaining rich data from a very small number of participants. The first of these concepts is 'theoretical sampling' (defined by Corbin and Strauss 2008, p.143). Snippets of conversation in the first interview are analysed for themes that then guide the conversation in the second interview. The same method is repeated between the second and the third, and the process continues in like fashion. This builds up, layer by layer, an understanding of the lived experience and social processes that operate. Subsequent interviews both guide the exploration and mitigate the impact of unusual views by individual participants.

The second of the two Grounded Theory concepts is known as 'theoretical saturation'. This is the point at which further interviews no longer add any new insights or knowledge to the findings or theories that are emerging. I recall that it was around the third or fourth interview that I developed the Perfect Storm Theory (Raffay 2012). I then tested and refined this in subsequent interviews and, by the time I reached the final interview, it was clear that the last two participants had agreed that was their experience and had little more to add to my enquiries.

Due to the disproportionate amount of time it took me to get ethical approval (and I did reasonably well compared with some researchers), I was left with little time to recruit and interview. My sample size of eight participants (of whom two withdrew) felt dangerously on the edge of viability. Thankfully, I did have enough participants to reach theoretical saturation.

The research process
Questions around the timing of the literature review

One of the most challenging issues I encountered was the suggestion by some advocates of Grounded Theory that conducting the literature review ahead of the interviews may result in any emergent theories being heavily influenced by earlier research. The alternative would be to have conducted the research and then later read the literature, but, in reality, my desire to conduct this particular piece of research emerged from my exposure to the literature. Furthermore, the ethics committees required evidence that I had engaged with current findings.

Choosing materials/literature (strengths of evidence)

I found myself somewhat bewildered by the amount of material written around spirituality and spiritual care. I quickly realised that I was not going to be able to exhaust the field within the timeframe of my Master's dissertation, and so would have to be selective. I could have done this by finding the most cited materials and quoting from them, though frequency of citation simply indicates popularity rather than necessarily quality. I therefore resorted to McSherry's (2007, pp.11–12) four domains of evidence in descending order of strength: (i) empirical; (ii) conceptual; (iii) professional/political; and (iv) personal. This model may not be suitable for all purposes, but it ensured that, wherever possible, I was drawing on evidence-based research rather than opinion. At the end of the day, however, I concluded that it is necessary to indicate understanding of the most cited texts.

As I read the literature, I was struck by the differences in what Corbin and Strauss (2008 pp.305–307) refer to as 'quality'. Many of the articles seemed to do little more than cover old ground, lacked any real engagement with the topic and offered little original thinking. Some, however, made altogether more interesting reading. They not only connected with experience but also informed the field (Corbin and Strauss 2008, p.305). I included some of the better articles for citation to evidence breadth of reading.

Database search

I searched eight databases using the search term: 'mental AND health AND spirit* AND (assessment OR tool)' and the date limiter '2004-current', the date being chosen because it offered a workable number of articles. I reduced the 275 results to 43, using the following inclusion criteria:

- use of Grounded Theory methodology or similar
- full text required (due to time constraints)
- relevance to study.

Modifying the search term to specify 'spiritual care' did not add any significant results. By using McSherry's (2007, pp.11–12) domains, I further reduced the 43 to nine studies.

Research ethics committees

I was told that seeking ethical approval for a Master's dissertation was not for the fainthearted, and am glad that I took the advice to heart. It was only when I committed myself to this that I fully appreciated the requirement to have (i) a fully worked out research proposal, (ii) research application and (iii) supporting papers, before approaching the ethics committees. I had imagined that I could bluff my way through, sharpening my thinking as I went through the interviews and presenting a nicely honed dissertation some months down the line. Not so. As a part-time student, it took me the best part of a month and frequent communication with my supervisor to get the documentation ready to apply.

In order to gain approval to conduct research with service users and staff, I applied through the online Integrated Research Ethics Application System. I did not find the website itself particularly complicated, but understanding the process and the various terms used was less than easy, as can be evidenced by a quick look at their help pages. My experience was that I had to wait about three weeks after submitting my application before I was given an interview. I was then asked for modifications, which caused further delay on an already tight deadline. As a result, I ended up with a short time frame to interview and write up my findings.

My experience highlighted for me the need to have a workable contingency plan in place so that I might have been able to complete my project if the unexpected had happened. One such plan might have been preparedness to conduct a literature review instead of field studies. Another might have been to save time on the ethics process by identifying a similar participant group not in NHS care (though this does not mean that I could have ignored ethical considerations). Another might have been to clarify conditions under which an extension could be obtained.

Research governance

I found it hard to understand the various research protocols and how they related to each other. My decision to conduct research with service users entailed a considerable amount of additional reading, and I found myself having to re-read the documentation on more than one occasion before I could make sense of it. For instance, I had to understand the difference between a chief and a principal investigator! I found it less than straightforward to grasp at what stage I could present my findings to the regional research committee and what many of the terms used actually meant. I also nearly failed to realise that I had to get insurance via the university.

Administering the research project

Funding

I found sourcing funding as well as managing funders and their expectations to be an important aspect of my project. Positively, funding provides a relationship that can be to mutual advantage in that it creates additional opportunities for dissemination of the findings. Negatively, it can influence what is researched or shape findings (Kendall *et al.* 2011). At the basic level, there is a reasonable obligation on the researcher to give regular updates to their funder(s) and to complete the project for which they have received the award. I did not experience any conflict of interest with my funders, but recognised that, under some circumstances, this could prove a very difficult matter indeed. My experience is that it is important to be realistic about funding and to avoid getting into a situation where time spent on seeking funding leaves insufficient time either to conduct the research itself or to maintain a reasonable social/family life.

Information technology

In the course of conducting my research, I found that effort spent refining my IT system (within reason) more than paid dividends. I particularly valued the security of having my data backed up securely, and I now use secure online backup as well as encrypted data sticks. On many occasions, I have ended up in a mess with different versions of documents – it is easy to do – so now have my laptop and desktop computers synchronised. I discovered that synchronisation is not the same as backup, the reason being that any mistake made is synchronised!

I may be an anxious fellow, but I also keep occasional printouts sorted in reverse date order for reference in case of total data meltdown. I use several passwords and have found it helpful to name a file with the first letter of the relevant password e.g. 'Filename (p)'. The reason for this is that I forgot the password for my data and sweated for a few days before I remembered it.

In order to keep tight version control of documents, I use the format: 'yyyy mm dd filename', an example of which is '2014 02 18 Dissertation'. The beauty of this system is that the files stack nicely in date order in the file explorer window. Dots and backslashes (\) are best avoided as they confuse the operating system.

Over the years, I have found scanning to be one of the trickiest processes to get right on a home computer. What is good nowadays is that it is generally possible to download a test version of the software before committing to it. Some of my peers have started scanning from their smart phones.

In terms of hardware, for creating documents such as a dissertation, I have found a keyboard far better than a touchscreen. I also bought myself a second-hand second monitor that cost very little and enables me to copy text from a source file into the document I am writing. In fairness, I had to replace the graphics card, but they are relatively inexpensive.

For interviewing, I bought a second-hand dictation machine on eBay in the knowledge that I could sell it on when it was finished with. A foot pedal was also useful but cost the best part of £100. On the advice of a friend, I used my mobile phone as a backup recording device.

Write-up – house styles

At times, I felt irritated by the precision required around punctuation, spelling, citations and so forth. However, it is commensurate with the level of precision that is required throughout the research process. Sloppiness around the research question or, even worse, around data security, risks not only a poor grade but also compromising research as a whole and reducing the ability of researchers to find willing participants.

I have found considerable differences between university style sheets, some of them being clear and others very confusing. I found it helpful to complement the style sheet with the appropriate style manual. I bought the next to latest version second-hand from abebooks.co.uk and saved myself lots of money! I could easily have become overwhelmed by the hundreds of recommendations, but I used it more as a reference book than as anything else.

Lifestyle

During the writing of this chapter, I have been planning a house move, my wife has had an operation and my father-in-law has passed away. Life does not conveniently come to a standstill to assist researchers in their enterprise! Having contingency plans was very useful, but keeping ahead of myself felt like the best safeguard against the unexpected.

I found regular exercise, healthy eating, sleeping and so on necessary to ensure I had the energy to remain focused and work effectively during the busy phases. In contrast to undergraduate essays, I found that research was more of a marathon than a sprint. Personally, it was important to me to keep a Sabbath rest, not just as a spiritual discipline but also because I found it made me more rather than less productive.

Impact of the research

Dissemination

It is easy to see one's horizon as the submission date, but, if a research project has value beyond obtaining a qualification, it is worth considering the matter of dissemination from the outset. If I am honest, I was aware of many opportunities in the course of the research project to cut corners or compromise on ethics, but these feelings were perhaps strongest when it came to dissemination. Part of me deeply desired to arrange for my work to be published in the most prestigious peer-reviewed journal I could get into. Though that may have advanced my potential academic career, there were many reasons why I did not choose this path. For a start, I have been significantly influenced by practical and liberation theology and am aware that research is shaped by power and politics. One person's perspective may be furthered at another's expense. Research ethics do not conclude when the data have been gathered, safely stored and analysed. A researcher has obligations to many people: to the participants; their funder (where appropriate); their peers; and their community, to name but a few. I decided that I would publish the core of my findings in the *Journal of Health Care Chaplaincy* (Raffay 2012) and in the *Journal of Nursing Management* (Raffay, 2013).

I wanted to allow chaplains and senior nurses to have access to my findings, as I believed that they would be best placed to serve the participants and bring about meaningful change.

I quickly became aware that, however good an article and however groundbreaking its content, I was unlikely to attract a readership if my title and abstract were not compelling. My favourite title: 'Are our mental health practices beyond HOPE?' (Raffay 2012) related to the HOPE assessment tool. I was also aware of the need for my abstract to contain keywords or phrases that would act as metadata for search engines.

Other outcomes

My research brought about significant changes in spiritual care practice in Sheffield Health and Social Care NHS Foundation Trust, where I was working at the time. These included getting spiritual care incorporated in care pathways and care clustering. The assessment tool that I produced (Raffay 2012) is starting to be used more widely in other mental health services, and I have just moved to Liverpool where I have taken up a post that combines research with clinical practice. I have recently obtained funding for a joint research project with Cardiff Centre for Chaplaincy Studies to co-produce a study into the possibilities of co-production in redesigning chaplaincy services. I am also in the first year of a professional doctorate at Durham University, where I am provisionally planning to co-produce research on the relationship between statutory mental health service providers and churches or faith communities. One small research project has had a huge impact on my life, and I hope that it will benefit others.

I have written at length about my previous research experience but hope now to co-produce any further work with service users (Faulkner 2004; Sweeney *et al.* 2009). I am convinced that this is not only the ethical way ahead but also the approach that is likely to be most fruitful in creating genuinely user-focused services (Francis 2013, p.87). I sincerely hope that, one day, ethics committees will require that all research involving mental health service users will be co-produced.

CHAPTER 11

How Secular is the NHS?

The Significance of Volunteers and Their Beliefs

Karen MacKinnon

Background

In 2009, media coverage followed the launch of University Hospital Southampton NHS Foundation Trust's Spiritual Care Policy, and included accusations of chaplains 'touting for business', with some seeing the move 'as a gross misuse of scarce National Health resources' (BBC 2009). This fed calls to remove healthcare chaplains from the publicly funded NHS (Christian 2011; NSS 2011), and articles in nursing journals that argued for the NHS remaining secular (Paley 2009). The debate continues around chaplaincy provision (BBC 2013; Davies 2013).

There is much evidence of secularisation in Britain. Attendance in traditional churches has declined (Brierley 2006; Mann 1853, cited in Warner 2010, pp.7–11). Those declaring themselves 'Christian' have declined by 18 per cent in the past decade, with a 9.5 per cent decline in people declaring a faith at all, and a 10 per cent increase in those stating that they have no religion (ONS 2012). The data are such that Brierley writes of the prospect of organised Christianity falling below the critical mass required to reproduce itself (Brierley 2000, p.28). Religion has less of an impact on people's day-to-day lives and public institutions than in the past, all of which leads Bruce to declare that 'Britain in 2030 will be a secular society' (Bruce 2003, p.62).

However, the situation is complex. Some point to Europe as being an exceptional case (Davie 2002), highlighting the rise of global religious movements (Davie 2002, pp.22, 139–140; Warner 2010, p.35) including fundamentalism (Armstrong 2000). Warner (2010, p.114) argues that, rather than signifying a retreat from the public square, pluralism and diversity of religion means that all religions may claim a voice in public life and points to the resilience of religious belief in a Europe that shows no 'appetite for absolute secularity' (2010, p.104). Many point to people's spirituality changing rather than dying, that people are 'believing differently' (Davie 2002, p.19) and that there is a 'spiritual revolution' taking place (Heelas and Woodhead 2005). As Taylor puts it, 'we are just at the beginning of a new age of religious searching, whose outcome no-one can foresee' (Taylor 2007, p.534).

My experience of staff and patients within the healthcare environment has been that, whilst the majority is not especially religious, most are open to spirituality in varying forms, especially in times of crisis. If one takes the popular understanding of 'secular' as antireligious (Nolan and Holloway 2014), the NHS seems to be an institution in which faith is respected and not overtly secular. Indeed, the Royal College of Nursing stresses that 'one cannot treat a person with dignity and respect unless attention is given to personal beliefs and values...however these may be defined, articulated and expressed' (McSherry 2011, p.6).

As a healthcare professional specialising in the area of spiritual care, the debate around secularism in the NHS aroused my keen interest. What do we mean by secularism or indeed spirituality? Are most people 'secular' or are they open to the spiritual aspects of humanity in all its myriad forms, especially in a context where matters of life and death are continually played out? The answers to such questions have a direct impact on healthcare chaplaincy and a wider impact on the spiritual and holistic care of patients, for the evolving nature of secularism and spirituality in Britain will determine the shape, or even existence, of spiritual care in the NHS in the future.

The research project design

As part of my MTh degree in healthcare chaplaincy at Cardiff University, I undertook a small research study of NHS volunteers in University Hospital Southampton NHS Foundation Trust (MacKinnon 2012). I wanted to explore how 'religious', 'spiritual' or 'secular' a group of NHS volunteers may be at a given moment; indeed, whether people would want to even classify themselves in these terms. The volunteers were a sizable group (1041), ethnically and religiously representative of the local population; they demonstrated a wide age range; and were engaged in a variety of tasks across the organisation. They seemed a reasonably representative group to survey.

A focus group approach was rejected for several reasons: (i) multiple groups would be needed to establish meaningful quantitative data; (ii) limitations of time; (iii) concern that focus groups would appeal to a vocal minority with strong religious/secular views; and (iv) the fact that people may not be totally honest if they knew that I, as researcher/group facilitator, am a chaplain. A survey sent to every hospital-registered volunteer seemed more likely to elicit honest views on a wider scale. After researching validated beliefs scales/ questionnaires, including that of King *et al.* (2006), I concluded that, in order to answer some of my particular questions arising from the literature review, I needed a bespoke survey.

The study was a mixed-method, cross-sectional survey. It was quantitative, in that it established factual data regarding how many participants agreed with certain statements. It was also qualitative, in that, by means of subsidiary questions, it explored the richer text of participants elaborating on their understanding of, and the meanings they gave to, these terms. Of the 1041 surveys sent out, 177 were returned completed within the deadline and by volunteers currently working for the Trust. These provided the raw data from which the following findings were obtained. Since the results of this survey represent a small percentage (17%) of the volunteer population, caution is needed when reaching conclusions. Nevertheless, these findings do shed important light on perceptions of spirituality, religion and secularity.

The research findings
Religiosity/secularity

The majority of questions were designed to ascertain whether the respondents retained traditional religious beliefs/practices, such as belief in God, prayer, worship attendance and some semblance of an enchanted worldview (Weber, Gerth and Wright Mills 1948, p.139), such as a belief in the supernatural, evil or destined purpose.

The findings reveal that a strong majority of the respondents (71%) believe in God. However, whilst 73 per cent of this group described a traditional understanding of God/Allah, the comments show much fluidity in interpretation, with the remainder of those believing in

God describing belief in a vaguer entity/power/something out there. Representative comments included:

I believe in the God revealed through the Bible, creation and the life, death and witness of Jesus Christ.

God or a higher power – definitely believe there is something but not necessarily the typical belief in God.

Having a choice of the above possibly shows that I believe in something, but maybe I can't pinpoint it to a particular form.

When asked to agree or disagree with the statement, 'I believe in life after death', the majority (53%) believed in life after death in some form or other, as seen in the comments:

Whilst I am not sure of what I believe happens after one dies, I don't believe that death is the end.

We either go to heaven or hell depending on the life we have led on earth.

Though others reported:

I think we just rot and push up daisies.

Of the respondents, 67 per cent agreed that, 'I sometimes pray' and 62 per cent agreed that, 'I sometimes feel a sense of the sacred when in a place of worship', describing this as:

Something big that I can't understand properly, but it touches every fibre of my spirit and myself.

A feeling of being somewhere special where I am in the presence of a greater force.

Whilst 65 per cent agreed with, 'I believe that there is a plan and purpose for my life', most believing this was directed by God or karma, others interpreted the question as plan and purpose being self-directed.

There was overall disagreement (62%) with the statement, 'Religion is irrelevant to my life.' Many felt that religion was not irrelevant because: (i) it was important to them; and (ii) it was important to others, therefore relevant to all. Others mentioned religion's moral and cultural heritage, as well as its negative influence. A few referred to morality without religion.

How can religion be irrelevant when hundreds of people all over the world are killing and dying at the behest of religious leaders who all profess to know what 'God' wants (Christians included).

Religion is present everywhere I go, in people I meet, patients that I care for. I…respect everyone's beliefs.

Religion is practised by the majority of the world, so it cannot be irrelevant.

Moral aspects of religion are not irrelevant.

Most of the respondents (48%) disagreed that they attended a place of worship regularly, a category frequently used as an indicator of secularisation. Of those who agreed they attended, the majority did so at least once a week, which suggests that the minority who attend a place of worship is very committed. Others expressed religious beliefs/practices whilst not being regular attendees.

You don't have to go to church to be a good Christian.

…not always have chance to go to church…but I pray regularly at home.

Opinions were much more evenly divided and uncertain around the statement, 'I believe in the supernatural,' than on any other question. Most defined 'supernatural' as inexplicable phenomena and ghosts, with many comments made around God/angels and also witchcraft/demons. Superhuman powers, aliens and 'spiritual' were also quoted with a number stating that they didn't know what to believe.

Supernatural forces are…those which cannot yet be explained by science.

To me it means 'something out there too big for me to understand'. The thought of it scares me so I try not to think about it very much.

I believe that there is a supernatural battle going on between God and Satan. God will win the battle, but Satan causes a lot of trouble at present.

I once lived in a house that had two ghosts there, and some of the things I experienced could not be explained other than by the word 'supernatural'.

Uncertainty around, 'I believe that there are supernatural evil forces in the universe,' were similarly expressed with comments split between references to personified evil, e.g. the devil, and purely human evil, with some stating a tension between feeling they ought to believe in supernatural evil but finding it difficult to do so.

We all make our own particular 'evil' in the world.

The thought of supernatural evil forces has been scaring me since I was a child; and in my religion God and evil have come hand in hand. I try to ignore the subject. (If not, I would be continuously terrified.)

As a Christian I should think that, but it is somehow difficult to accept.

Despite 80 per cent of respondents associating themselves with a faith, only 42 per cent agreed with the statement, 'I consider myself to be a religious person.' The following comments reveal the ambiguity:

Religious is not just going to church but putting faith into action.

My religion is looking after any human who needs help from me.

I have a faith that informs my moral sense of right and wrong and informs my daily actions and sense of self.

Pigeon-holed.

I see myself as spiritual than religious [sic.]. I see religious as being a member of a set religion... I am interested in all though cannot commit to one in particular... I like the fact that I can remain neutral and enjoy it all.

I'm not sure I'd want to be identified as a religious person. 'Religion' is responsible for a lot of pain in the world.

Yet neither did the majority of respondents consider themselves to be secular, with 40 per cent disagreeing with the statement, 'I consider myself to be a secular person.' There was a significant number (28%) who neither agreed nor disagreed, and the comments revealed that many did not understand what the term meant. Those who did, envisaged some separation from religion: some expressing it as being somehow 'worldly', wavering as to whether this was a positive or negative thing; others understood the term as relating to a 'religious' working in the world (voicing an early meaning of the word), and disagreed with the statement because they were not in holy orders. The following comments are representative:

Worldly and not religious.

The state being separate from religion.

I understand that secular means getting rid of any expression of God in society.

This is a difficult question to answer since all of us live in and cope with a secular world. To that extent we are all secular, however strong our religious side of life is. But we generally use secular to refer to the rational world in which religious faith has no part, and if that definition is accepted I am not a secular person.

Parts of me are.

Spirituality

Some questions were designed to explore spirituality as distinct from religion. Whilst the comments show that it is difficult to disentangle the two, the responses give an indication of what people mean by spirituality and evidence Reed's (1992) definition of spirituality as:

the propensity to make meaning through a sense of relatedness to dimensions that transcend the self…[that] may be experienced intrapersonally (as a connectedness within oneself), interpersonally (in the context of others and the natural environment) and transpersonally (referring to a sense of relatedness to the unseen, God or power greater than the self). (Reed 1992, p.350)

Of the respondents, 47 per cent agreed with the statement that, 'At least once in my life, I have had what I consider to be a spiritual experience.' This was explained by religious experiences describing answered prayers, feelings of God's presence and protection, as well as broader descriptions of post-bereavement and near-death experiences, powerful dreams, identifying with nature and strong feelings.

The majority agreed that, 'A deep sense of connectedness with nature and/or the Universe is important to me,' though 28 per cent neither agreed nor disagreed. Comments described connection with various natural aspects – the sea and countryside being mentioned most – alongside descriptions of feelings nature engendered within them, notably calmness, peace and wonder. Many mentioned nature bringing them closer to the creator, others the responsibility humanity has for the planet.

After a loss it becomes very important for me to connect with the beauty of nature.

Through nature I find God.

When I feel peaceful, content, I feel closest to Nature. It is important for me to feel this as I strive to find my true self and the feeling of all of us and everything around us is connected.

An overwhelming majority of respondents (81%) agreed that, 'A deep sense of connectedness to others is important to me.' The comments revealed that family/friends are the most important relationships, with a strong emphasis on socialising and helping those in need. Equally, a strong sense of well-being and sense of purpose was generated through this connection.

Reaching out to others and having them connect with me is very important. Empathy with others enhances my spiritual wellbeing.

The majority of respondents (64%) also agreed that, 'A deep sense of connectedness within myself *is important to me.*' Most identified this as accepting oneself and as necessary for one to help others, as well as being important in providing a sense of purpose.

Knowing yourself and being happy in your own skin.

Only at times when I am connected within myself I feel spiritually elevated and at peace.

Especially when I help others, I feel that 'inner' connection. It's who I am… It makes me 'whole'.

The majority of respondents agreed with the statement, 'I consider myself to be a spiritual person,' with 24 per cent being undecided. Whilst most comments linked spiritual to religious aspects, others linked the word to relating to the non-material world, connection with others, self and nature.

Inspired and connected to the 'divine', which can be different for each one of us.

…things that touch the spirit: music, art, nature, people etc.

A knowledge that there is a 'being' (God) existing in my life who looks after me and who I can turn to in need.

strong connectedness with the world…nature, other people and with themselves.

Spiritual and religious care in the NHS

The final survey questions are particularly pertinent to the secularisation debate and were designed to establish how important volunteers feel spiritual and religious care is in the NHS.

An overwhelming majority of respondents (72%) agreed with the statement, 'I think that spiritual and religious care is important, especially when people are experiencing difficult situations.' Almost all of the 123 respondents who commented stated that this care brought comfort, consolation and hope for people. Others added the proviso that this was important but shouldn't be imposed.

> *While I may be an atheist, I believe that for those who are religious and experiencing difficult situations, it is very important.*

> *I believe that patients have a right to expect not only their physical and mental needs but also their spiritual and religious needs to be met in hospital.*

> *When any of us are going through difficult moments our need is for love and hope, warmth, trust – all that is found in spiritual care of others.*

> *We are holistic people, and our physical health is closely linked to our mental and spiritual health.*

Whilst 24 per cent were uncertain, the majority of respondents agreed that, 'I think that it's part of the NHS's role to provide spiritual and religious care.' For those who agreed, this was seen to be an important part of holistic care, giving comfort and aiding the recovery process. A number added the caveat that it should be provided only for those who want this. Of those who disagreed, it was stressed either that the NHS was for physical/mental care only, or that the churches should provide this care.

> *The NHS provides medical care. It is not in the business of providing religious and spiritual care. That is the business of religious organisations.*

> *Everybody is an individual, and if the NHS believe in providing individualised care, then they must take into account the needs of people, even if spiritual or religious.*

> *If it contributes to a person's wellbeing, then yes.*

> *Not enough funding for medical services, let alone religious care.*

> *People are body and soul and real healing can be found in the loving treatment and care of both.*

An overwhelming majority (81%) agreed that, 'If I or a loved one was in hospital and in distress, I might value spiritual support,' listing the kinds of support wanted, primarily listening, emotional and prayer support.

> *Someone to open up to who is not medical. Someone who can empathise with my fears and needs beyond medical care.*

> *In the 'hustle and bustle' of hospitals, somebody to really 'listen' to you can be very valued!*

> *Someone with whom one could pray.*

> *A visit by a chaplain of my own faith.*

Discussion

For this NHS group, the findings showed that whilst secularisation was evidenced in terms of decline in religious attendance and less belief in the supernatural, the position is much less evidenced in terms of religious beliefs. The majority expressed belief in God, life after death and prayed. Yet the respondents did not appear to want to be labelled. Around half of those who had a faith did not want to be described as 'religious', nor did the vast majority identify themselves with being 'secular'. Of the three terms considered, people seemed most at ease around the word 'spiritual'.

For many, their beliefs were fluid, containing orthodox understandings alongside their own subjective interpretations, as can be seen from the following comments:

> *I see myself as spiritual than religious [sic.]. I see religious as being a member of a set religion… I am interested in all though cannot commit to one in particular… I like the fact that I can remain neutral and enjoy it all.*

> *Religious means following a religion – mainstream or your personal one.*

> *I believe in a higher power and try to live my life as a good person. I don't necessarily agree with the teachings and dogma of the faith I was born in, and I am open to other ideas.*

The comments suggest that beliefs are changing and evolving, with less reliance on received teaching as in the past, and more on picking and mixing from a smorgasbord of spiritualities and faith systems, choosing whatever seems most appropriate for the individual.

The humanist definition of 'secularist' is someone who believes:

that laws and public institutions…should be neutral as between alternative religions and beliefs. Almost all humanists are secularists, but religious believers may also take a secularist position which calls for freedom of belief, including the right to change belief and not to believe. Secularists seek to ensure that persons and organisations are neither privileged nor disadvantaged by virtue of their religion or lack of it… The word 'secularism' was once used to describe a non-religious world view generally but this meaning is now very old fashioned. (BHA 2014)

On this basis, it seems that the respondents largely take a secularist position in terms of freedom of religious belief, yet react against being considered secular – this being interpreted by them as being non- or even antireligious. Overall, the respondents' comments displayed an openness and tolerance to those of all beliefs and none, which perhaps reflects not just their attitude, but that of the NHS in general.

To healthcare chaplains, the findings in this survey will not come as a surprise. It connects with their daily experience. Many of the patients they support declare that they are not religious and yet during the pastoral encounter report to the chaplain their belief in God, life after death and request prayer. What we do find in this survey – apart from evidence of these beliefs – is that not only do this group of volunteers strongly believe spiritual/religious care is important for others, they also believe that they might appreciate this care themselves if they were in hospital, that it should be provided by the NHS, and they also tell us what this care should look like. They express the importance of having someone to listen to them, give them emotional support, pray with them, make them feel valued; to explore the meaning of suffering, life, death with; to hold their hand, comfort, give them the sacraments – all in an accepting non-judgemental way. Connectedness with others is a key component of their spirituality, as well as with nature and within themselves, confirming the definition of spirituality as 'the aspect of humanity that refers to the way individuals seek and express meaning and purpose, and the way they experience their connectedness to the moment, to self, to others, to nature, and to the significant or sacred' (Puchalski and Ferrell 2010, p.25). We find evidence that these matters are important and perhaps particularly so during sickness. They confirm the validity of chaplaincy practice.

Whilst the survey was a local one, it does not seem unreasonable to suggest that the views of the respondents may be typical of the general population. However, to establish this would require further research.

Nonetheless, in considering what caring for the whole person might mean in an age of both secularisation and spiritual evolution, the survey findings have significance for spiritual/religious care provision in the NHS. The majority in the survey did not describe themselves as 'religious', yet they clearly felt that generic spiritual – as well as religious – care was important in their healthcare. People have beliefs that are important to them, and this fact has implications for those involved in admission processes and care pathways. The fact that people hold a variety of deeply held beliefs needs to be borne in mind, irrespective of whether they declare a faith on admission – waiting only until near death to support these needs, which is the usual trigger for spiritual care referrals, is not good enough spiritual care. Equally, accounting only for the local *religious* population, means the majority may be denied the spiritual care they might greatly value. Skill and sensitivity are required to ensure the right questions are asked, and staff confidence and education need to be raised to ensure that all who want it can access this support as part of their patient experience.

Caring for the whole person is complex, and NHS chaplains are well aware of the flexibility and fluidity of beliefs: the 'non-religious' patient requesting prayer; the 'Christian' believing in reincarnation. If secularisation continues, chaplains may experience an increase in hybrid beliefs and various spiritualities, with an attendant need to find connectedness, meaning and hope. Chaplains may have to refine their skills, relying less on delivering 'routine' liturgical care, Holy Communion, etc., and more on developing new, accessible liturgies embracing these spiritualities (e.g. developing creative and meaningful memorial services for non-religious staff, baby funerals, blessings for young parents of no faith or mixed faith traditions). This spiritual evolution, or 'revolution' (Heelas and Woodhead 2005), is a critical component of contemporary chaplaincy interaction.

Conclusion

It would seem from both the survey and from my professional experience of working within the NHS, that whilst some elements of secularisation are evident, religious faith in Britain is certainly not dead. The situation does not appear terminal (Warner 2010, p.182); rather, spirituality is evolving and the NHS is keen to engage with this evolution through its policies, frameworks and evidence-based practice. The ethos seems to be that of not only taking a secularist position in terms of tolerating freedom of religious belief, but indeed of respecting faith.

It is an interesting time for spiritual care as we move into an age that, on some levels, is regarded as secular, in that religion ceases to occupy the dominant space in the public sphere which it once held, yet which contrarily seems also to be a time of spiritual evolution – perhaps growing outside of what some (Jamieson 2002; Jamieson, McIntosh and Thompson 2006) might call the 'faith limiting environment' of the churches.

The NHS cares for the nation's citizens with regards to their health. If those citizens prefer holistic care, then provision must be made for the spiritual and religious care of citizens who prefer that it be available to them. If the majority does not require spiritual and religious care, it will disappear naturally, without need for media campaigns. This survey shows that for one group of NHS volunteers at least, this is far from the current situation, and, pending further research, hints that our secular NHS nevertheless, respects faith and spirituality in its caring of the whole person.

A personal view

Caring for the whole person in an age of secularisation also necessarily involves engaging with what is meant by 'secularism' and 'secular'. Certainly the survey respondents demonstrated confusion over whether they should be 'worldly' or not in response to the specific question on whether they considered themselves to be secular. Here perhaps is a role for theologians as well as chaplains as one explores reclaiming the word 'secular' and not leaving it solely to fundamentalist antireligionists. Personally, I consider myself to be a secular priest, and by that mean something more than simply being a priest working in a secular environment. For me, it is about resisting the divorce between the earthly and divine and rather finding a synthesis, finding the divine in the world, connecting the sacred and secular. Resisting being confined to the narrowly religious box, 'set apart' on some 'holy mission', but instead embracing the human kaleidoscope of spirituality, as one healthcare professional amongst others, engaged in exploring how we can best support people in a holistic and life affirming way. I am both secular (of this age, world), with an interest and love for the non-religious in my world, as well as a person of faith in something beyond this world. The God I believe in is not confined to any religious faith, but is to be found as much in the world as in any church. The healthcare chaplain as secular priest is uniquely placed, both literally and symbolically to represent the human and divine. A symbol of the importance of respect for all human life, dignity, beliefs and values, as well as pointing to the transcendent, in whatever form that may take.

CHAPTER 12

Observing, Recording and Analysing Spiritual Care in an Acute Setting

Rodney Baxendale

Chaplaincy: Loved but not justified?

Most healthcare chaplains working in the NHS are aware of contradictory forces at work daily, or when their departments are challenged to justify the size of their teams, or in the annual round of budget examination. First, they are generally liked, with much individual appreciation; second, the Finance Director will say, with a sad smile, that that is no longer enough, and chaplains need to justify the extent of their existence.

Within the wider context of healthcare chaplaincy, awareness of this tension is apparent in the 'Caring for the spirit' project, designed to support the development of healthcare chaplaincy in the UK, led initially by the South Yorkshire Workforce Development Confederation (2003). Such awareness is seen particularly in the encouragement given, as part of 'Caring for the spirit' to chaplains in the UK to develop a 'minimum data-set' (MDS). As discussed in Chapter 5, part of the rationale for the development of an MDS, alongside the benefits for good practice, is that data should be monitored: 'To establish best use of resources'; and 'To provide value for money' (South Yorkshire Workforce Development Confederation 2004, p.2).

Similar concerns to provide an evidential base for both good practice and financial worth are to be seen in the current transatlantic debate about whether chaplaincy should work with an outcomes-based model of chaplaincy (see, e.g. Handzo *et al*. 2014). A key question that emerges from the whole debate, and the aim of engaging in the quantification and collection of data on all manner of chaplaincy activities, including encounters, call-outs, referrals and a range of specific duties (South Yorkshire Workforce Development Confederation 2004), is how such mapping can be conducted in such a way that the depth of spiritual care provided by chaplains is not obscured in the process.

This chapter presents one approach, in a particular context, to the quantitative mapping of chaplaincy that seeks to avoid the pitfall just identified, as well as giving the hospital's Finance Director a happier smile! The project (Baxendale 2010) had the aim of gathering data about the nature of our activities; in other words, more data than simple visit numbers. Though tallies of visits conducted convinced most that our department was busy, that was never quite the detail that was needed: what were we busy at, and how skilled were we in our busyness?

The task was to devise a method of collecting information during the ordinary working day, by chaplains and volunteers alike that could present a quantifiable picture to outside enquirers, and be valuable to the department itself, helping to understand our work, and provide us with targets for improving our techniques, our usage of personnel. While I was doing this I was also hopeful that something could be produced that started to identify something of the *quality* of our work. In one sense, this approach is precisely in keeping with that of the 'Caring for the spirit' MDS proposal, in which the MDS is just that, a minimum – a foundation for developing further understanding of spiritual care (South Yorkshire Workforce Development Confederation 2004).

A survey of a given week's activity gave focus to the project, and enabled the department to 'own' the project.

The centrepiece of the project was the production of a question sheet to capture the detail of each incident experienced by department members – the research instrument. The results were analysed by a computer program already licensed to the Trust (SNAP9). The document was designed to be very flexible, capable of any enquiry I might make, and able to be quickly amended to examine a single area deeply, or everything we did more superficially.

This chapter considers: first, the research process, complete with teething troubles; second, examples of the data derived from the survey, with some of the insights gained, as an indication of its potential; and third, the wider value of this model for chaplaincy, to encourage others to work towards the holy grail of devising methods that will display the qualitative benefits of chaplaincy in ways that will convince the most demanding of quantitative enquirers.

Sequence of the project

The project plan was developed in consultation with other hospital departments, whose initial friendly incomprehension gave way to equally friendly cooperation. The main stages of the project were:

1. seeking ethical approval
2. developing the research instrument and running a pilot day
3. conducting and managing the survey week
4. data input and analysis.

Seeking ethical approval

The main question in relation to this project was whether it constituted 'research', as understood by the NHS, or 'service evaluation' and therefore 'audit'. The central criterion is whether a project will result in new, generalisable data, or simply present a survey of current or historic practice. This project was defined as audit, which required less stringent approval (from an Audit Panel) – nevertheless it required justification, itself valuable.

Developing the research instrument

Development of the research instrument, or survey document (Figure 12.1a and b) was core to the project's aim and methodology, and centred around 'the pastoral encounter', repeated countless times in every chaplaincy. This survey document was going to be used repeatedly and needed to harvest considerable amounts of information from each event, without impeding the work itself.

The survey document needed to be definite in its descriptions of subject areas, and to be answerable overwhelmingly by tick box. The following six central decisions were taken, arising out of the consultative design process. First, a decision was taken on the type of encounters to be recorded – administrative, a non-pastoral (general) conversation, or a pastoral encounter. Second, it was decided to permit free text descriptions where necessary. Third, it became clear that the form needed to be capable of swift completion, to minimise interference with the work. Fourth, the form had to allow for swift comparative analysis between various sub-groups of respondents, by a computer analysis program. Fifth, it had to allow for indexing of respondents, to equalise their comments and assessments. Sixth, the form needed to accommodate respondents' judgements and evaluations, in addition to numerical data.

Of these considerations, the most key in carrying out the survey were speed and ease of completion: the pastoral encounters were genuine, and interrupting the process for form-filling would have been destructive.

In broad terms, the survey document developed into a double-sided sheet, with five main sections, each kept as brief and uncluttered as possible, comprising the following sections:

- Introductory material: date and time, identity of the respondent, and length of the pastoral encounter (Q1–Q5).

- Definition of the functional type of the reported encounter and identification of subject areas (Q6–Q8).

- A 'judgement' section, inviting responses on various success ratings of the encounter (Q9–Q12). These questions invited the respondents to make subjective judgements about various aspects of their reported encounter. Respondents were invited to judge encounters by a short series of ranges: from 'mundane' to 'specialist-spiritual'; from 'simple' to 'complex'; from 'unsuccessful encounter' to 'successful encounter'; and from 'rapport not established' to 'rapport established'.

- A section identifying the protagonists in the encounter, place and method of communication (Q13–Q18). The questions in this section were to establish factual information about the encounter: Where did it take place? Who was it with? Who initiated the encounter? Was the encounter planned, anticipated or fortuitous? In particular, Question 18 established whether the encounter was face-to-face, or via telephone or email. These parameters proved instructive, especially about the geographical reach of the chaplaincy, its proactive nature and the dynamic character of its encounters.

Anonymous 'discriminator boxes' were added at the end of the document, to be completed by the results compiler. These were to permit further analysis, allowing categorisations of the respondents to be added post-completion. The significance and completion of these boxes were exclusively in my hands (they could be varied to suit the needs of each survey).

- Box A: male or female.

- Box B: age groups, defined as 30–40, 41–50, 51–60, 60+. (There are no members of the department at present younger than 30.)

- Box C: clergy or lay.

- Box D: 'optimism' index. This was a primitive attempt to separate responses by an assessment of the innate tendency of individual respondents to over- or under-assess the success of encounters. It was determined by a meeting of the core team of chaplains, and was defined as follows: 'not known', 'very optimistic', 'fairly optimistic', 'neutral', 'fairly pessimistic' and 'very pessimistic'.

- Box E: time in minutes of encounter. Most encounters lasted less than ten minutes at the bedside, but longer visits tended to presage some deepening of the subject matter, or less frequently, a communication problem. Very long encounters, of 45 minutes or more, were of particular significance, as they inferred a strong contribution from the patient or family.

Many of the more valuable responses were of course subjective judgements: the nub of future projects may well be to pin these judgements down with external criteria; shadowing members of the department might be needed, as long as their presence did not compromise the exchanges. This might refine the subjective nature of the judgement, if never entirely removing it. The work on the optimism factor in the study suggested that even the most optimistic members of the team were quite clear-sighted about the success of their encounters.

There remains a wide spectrum of opinion of what constitutes 'success' in a pastoral encounter: achieving rapport is itself a success, but assessing successful outcomes is more problematic. The focus in this study is clearly on perceptions of immediate success. The most significant use of this information was in determining whether the innate optimism of particular individuals skewed their personal success estimates: Table 12.4 displays the resulting data, and would suggest that it did not.

Event
Number

Survey use only

Chaplains

Plymouth Hospitals NHS
NHS Trust

Department of Pastoral & Spiritual Care

Survey Recording Sheet 2010 - PLEASE USE A NEW SHEET FOR EACH EVENT

Q1 Date:

Q2 Your first initial and surname please:

Q3 Event Start Time:

Q4 Event End Time:

Q5 Was this Event or Encounter..?

Administrative? .... □ Go to Q6

A non-pastoral (general) conversation? .... □ Go to Q6

A pastoral encounter? .... □ Go to Q7

Q6 Describe the subject of the conversation briefly

Go to Q9

Q7 If it was a pastoral conversation, please identify the areas covered: tick all boxes that are relevant:

General topical chat .... □
Chat becoming more personal .... □
Personal distress .... □
Personal spirituality .... □
Loneliness .... □
Personal confession .... □
Prayer .... □
End of Life .... □
Bereavement .... □
Anger management .... □
Communion .... □
Anointing .... □
Rejoicing .... □
Referral to own faith community ..... □
Naming and Blessing .... □
Baptism .... □
Scripture-reading .... □

Q8 If another subject area, please describe briefly:

Q9 How would you assess the following aspects of this encounter: mark the box which reflects your answer most closely

Mundane	Less Mundane	Partly spiritual	Specially Spiritual
□	□	□	□

Figure 12.1a Recording document

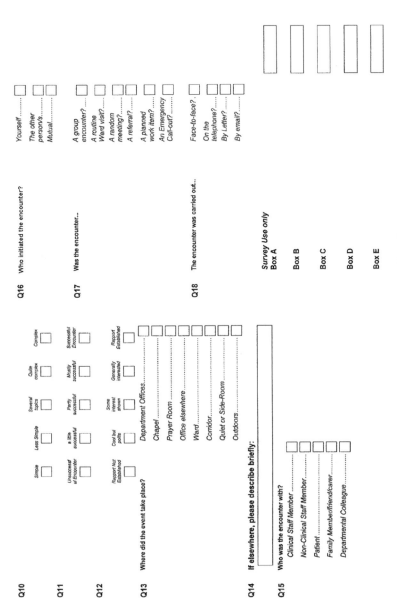

Q10 Who initiated the encounter?

Yourself.......... ☐
The other person's.......... ☐
Mutual.......... ☐

Q11 Was the encounter...

A group encounter? ☐
A routine Ward visit? ☐
A random meeting? ☐
A referral? ☐

A planned work item? ☐
An Emergency Call-out? ☐

Q18 The encounter was carried out...

Face-to-face? ☐
On the telephone? ☐
By Letter? ☐
By email? ☐

Survey Use only
Box A
Box B
Box C
Box D
Box E

Q10 Who initiated the encounter?

Q11

	Simple	Less Simple	Several topics	Quite complex	Complex
	☐	☐	☐	☐	☐

	Unsuccessful Encounter	a little successful	Partly successful	Mostly successful	Successful Encounter
	☐	☐	☐	☐	☐

Q12

	Cool but polite	Some interest shown	Generally interested	Rapport Established
Rapport Not Established	☐	☐	☐	☐

Q13 Where did the event take place?

Department Offices.......... ☐
Chapel.......... ☐
Prayer Room.......... ☐
Office elsewhere.......... ☐
Ward.......... ☐
Corridor.......... ☐
Quiet or Side-Room.......... ☐
Outdoors.......... ☐

Q14 If elsewhere, please describe briefly:

Q15 Who was the encounter with?

Clinical Staff Member.......... ☐
Non-Clinical Staff Member.......... ☐
Patient.......... ☐
Family Member/friend/carer.......... ☐
Departmental Colleague.......... ☐

Figure 12.1b Back page of recording document

As part of the development of the research instrument, four different focus groups were run, corresponding to the main personnel groups within the department: chaplains, both employed and honorary; pastoral team members; administration volunteers; and weekend volunteers. The purpose of the groups was essentially to validate the content of the draft survey document. This was done by getting focus groups to establish the main activities in which they were engaged within their chaplaincy work. This allowed the categories deployed in questions five and seven of the survey document, in particular, to be checked against current practice. The occasion also proved to be a valuable team-building exercise, particularly for the volunteer groups, and an opportunity to describe the project more fully, although this was done on completion of the structured research exercise described previously.

A pilot survey day was planned to assess the ease of use and practicality of the document and method, to determine how briefing should be framed and to establish how the whole experience might be received by patients, staff and the visitors themselves. The day was carried out without prior warning, to avoid uncharacteristic absenteeism. Twelve documents were completed and the participants were interviewed on the experience.

It was agreed that completing the document was not irksome or intrusive, though keeping it out of sight was important. Queries from participants ranged from enquiries as to how to distinguish between a non-pastoral (general) conversation, and an administrative encounter; criteria for assessing the nature of a conversation – 'mundane' was construed in one instance as a pejorative adjective, and in another as 'obscure'. The term 'specialist-spiritual' replaced 'spiritual', to differentiate discussions of spiritual distress or fulfilment from discussions of emotional matters. Minor changes to the document were then made.

The most important decision made as a result of the pilot day was to place the consent and information process at the *end* of encounters, rather than at the start – the conversations remained authentic, and could be easily excluded from the study if consent was not given.

Conducting and managing the survey

The week chosen for the survey was arbitrary, dictated more by my availability than any other consideration; it was the first available week when I could be on duty every day to supervise and brief those concerned. In any event, any week would have its own distinctive features, but the features themselves would not alter the basic building bricks of the department's activities: visiting, counselling, providing spiritual support would always be present. From a personal viewpoint, it was exceedingly draining, but satisfying.

The survey was held from 08:00 on Monday 29 March 2010 to 07:59 on Monday 5 April 2010. Coincidentally, this was Holy Week and Easter, but the life of the hospital is little driven by the liturgical year, other than a slight overall reduction in both inpatients and clinics. The week was not announced publicly, nor were members of the department other than the core chaplain team informed in advance. This was to discourage large-scale absenteeism, and worked overwhelmingly: only one member of the core team did not participate in the reporting procedure, owing to pressure of visiting obligations. This absence from the record did not distort the survey, as any week might contain the absence on leave or study of an individual team member.

Briefing of those taking part was as individual as possible, and took place as each arrived for duty. Most had already taken part in the focus group exercise, and were to some extent prepared by that for the survey. Each member of the department was individually briefed about the use of consent and information sheets and the completion of activity logs, and invited to choose a representative selection of encounters for completion using the survey document. There was a workmanlike feel about the process, which included a sense that all members of the department were taken seriously as colleagues, which was heartening.

Respondents were invited to record a representative selection of their day's events. Though items thought to be 'interesting' or 'significant' should figure, the 'dull' and 'routine' should also be included. Other criteria were that events that were assessed as less successful should be included, lest all events were recorded as wholly successful. There is no denying that this is subjective: on another occasion the rules could be changed, and every event could be recorded, or only encounters of a particular type. Although the decision not to record all encounters weakens the data as a quantitative indicator of the overall scope of the department's work, the decision allowed department members to focus on recording data relating to the nature of the encounters. And the size of the sample still allowed for a range of quantifications (see later).

Other than an explanation of the process, it was stressed that the exercise was a departmental self-examination. It was not an assessment of individuals or the work; merely a record of what actually happened.

Some 50 different individuals were involved in entering encounters into the survey, which contained 141 entries, spread between the four groups: chaplains, pastoral team members, administrative staff and weekend volunteers. Chaplains, working throughout the study week, thereby gained most practice in manipulating the form, and so produced the most 'expert' work. Pastoral team members typically work one session a week, and hence only had one opportunity to use the document. However, there were only five spoilt papers, and these were solely due to failure to complete page two of the document. This represented a spoilage rate for the survey of 3.4 per cent.

The design of the survey document appeared to be validated by the experience of the participants, as was the completion of consent forms following encounters: speed of completion was achieved, together with a lack of interruption of the chaplaincy tasks themselves by completing the document. For most members of the department the burden was relatively light. The survey document was designed to be capable of use by any member of the department, and this proved to be so. This is important, as generating an overall desire 'to do research' makes each successive project easier to complete, with a high level of willing cooperation.

Discussion around the design of the document generated a small array of positive comments. Although a 'tick box' format was initially viewed as inadequate for the recording of such a complex task, actual experience changed people's minds. The speed with which it could be completed was seen as 'practical' – the same comment was heard concerning the consent and information sheets, administered after the encounters. Terms like 'anger management' (Q7) and 'mundane' (Q9) needed further explanation, and the presence of a box in Q17 entitled 'a random meeting' engendered an unexpected theological dispute – opinions varied as to whether such a thing existed in the divine economy!

The need for respondents to identify themselves gave rise to comment, when combined with the previous assurance that anonymity would be preserved. The explanation that it had a bearing on the contents of the boxes sufficed, together with the assurance that names would remain in the computer, and not form any part of the finished results. Once the briefings were completed, there were no refusals to take part.

Data input and analysis

Practical problems centred around the limitations on manpower for the processing of the resultant data: the writer was a staff of one: data entry into the SNAP9 analysis program could only be attempted out of working hours, as only a single-user licence is held by the Trust, and only a specific computer could be employed by a user.

Once data entry was complete, the program could be interrogated for total numbers for different categories and further sifting. Broadly, two distinct types of enquiries were employed:

1. audit-type questions, giving totals for particular activities or groups of individuals, subject-matter questions, and so on

2. discriminating questions, exploring possible correlation between one set of data and another (sections of the staff, age groups, clergy or lay, and so on), looking for trends and patterns behind the overall totals.

Audit questions in general have proved useful in defining chaplaincy 'busyness' to external enquiry; discriminating questions appear most useful in stimulating internal conversation, planning and thought, and lines for future enquiry.

The process threw up high quantities of usable subject area data, and is a good basis for training syllabus material. A simple reading of the subjects covered in encounters gives a vivid picture of the looking-glass world of healthcare chaplaincy: a patient's anxiety over their pet parrot's temporary home; faith issues versus acknowledgement of illness symptoms; mastectomy pain relief on a patient's 50th wedding anniversary. A complete list was included in Baxendale (2010, pp.55ff).

The sheer quantity of data realisable from the computer analysis program was truly staggering, and not all of it strictly helpful. The crucial task was to decide on the questions to be asked and to instruct the program to correlate the relevant sets of data to reveal the patterns beneath. This was time-consuming, but became increasingly productive as proficiency with the program improved. The Trust's training department was of great assistance in focusing attention, when I was immobilised by the sheer volume of information and possible enquiries.

The questions asked varied from the degree of perceived success achieved by the various categories of staff, through setting the complexity of the encounter against perceived success, to more apparently mundane matters such as who initiated most pastoral encounters. However, almost any combination of data was possible: the subject areas covered by chaplains compared with pastoral team members; length of encounter; the relative perceived success rates of males and females, old and young.

Though the survey document had proved to be appropriately brief, it was only employed for selected events in each day as it might become onerous if used for *every* encounter. One in three of the 141 documents submitted required the use of subject area boxes to explain subjects covered, and any revision would therefore require greater breadth of subject areas, rather than less.

Findings

This section of the chapter demonstrates the varying types of findings that were derived from this particular project. Although I was concerned with establishing a method for displaying the department's activities in general, as indicated earlier in the chapter, a key concern was pursuing the quality of encounters.

Questions 7 and 8: Subject areas covered in pastoral encounters

Answers to these over-arching questions painted a detailed portrait of the department's activity: chaplains' conversations clustered around distress, spirituality and prayer, with end-of-life concerns figuring in 5.9 per cent of their encounters; pastoral team encounters are more evenly spread, with a far greater proportion of encounters beginning routinely, and then evolving into spirituality. This would be consistent with chaplains' visits being often the result of referrals to them; in contrast to the ice-breaking quality of pastoral team visiting. Pie charts were constructed for each group, producing a very detailed picture of the conversations (Baxendale 2010, pp.53–54).

The different groups picked up different emotions: for example, loneliness was detected by the visitors more frequently, as an underlying emotion informing patients' coping abilities. They frequently had more time to devote at the bedside than chaplains responding to urgent calls. Prayer was more frequently requested from chaplains, but also from the weekend teams, with unsuccessful worship-attenders (those declaring a wish to attend worship, but then declining when volunteers arrive to collect them).

In the short term these results emphasised where the demands really lay, rather than our preconceptions. In the longer term, they provided a list of training needs, and much content for future reflective sessions.

Questions 9 and 10: Qualities of the encounter

Turning to the questions surrounding matters of 'success' in encounters, it is at this point that assessments became more subjective: though I believe these results speak sound good sense, the future lies in establishing closer methods of indexing the responses from individual respondents, as much as the more tenuous search for objective definitions of the word 'success' itself. A comment frequently heard from members of the department was that all that was possible was an assessment of the encounter itself, rather than the ultimate resolution. If we come from a bedside having empathetically connected with a patient in distress, engaged in a dialogue at a profound level, then that encounter was a success in our terms – whether we consequently shortened the patient's inpatient time is perhaps always going to be beyond the far side of research. A further area for future research would correlate chaplaincy team responses with responses sought from patients, as to their perceptions and evaluations of their encounters with chaplains.

Both chaplains and the pastoral team categorised their encounters as increasingly spiritual across the range: however, the pastoral team assessed the complexity as one grade less than Chaplains: only 8.2 per cent of their encounters were assessed as specialist-spiritual, compared with 53.3 per cent for chaplains. This reflects the general operating practice of referrals to chaplains on situations assessed previously by the pastoral team as difficult or long term. Chaplains did not interpret any of their encounters as mundane: the spiritual component was always deemed to be present.

The pattern observed in Q9 is repeated in Q10 when the question of perceived complexity is addressed: the pastoral team consider themselves involved in somewhat less complex encounters than chaplains – they also seem more ready to evaluate a significant proportion of their encounters (26.2%) as more or less simple.

The pastoral team determined that 41 per cent of their encounters involved 'several topics', a category designed to characterise an encounter as hybrid: originally a social conversational exchange (a 'Plymouth Argyle' conversation), which might be wide-ranging, might hint at deeper concerns or emotions, but did not develop into an overtly spiritual conversation, probably earning it a 'complex' rating.

Question 11: Assessment of success

Table 12.1 Assessment of success results

Q11: Success	N	Unsuccessful encounter	A little successful	Partly successful	Mostly successful	Successful encounter
Combined count	139	3 (2.2%)	4 (2.9%)	13 (9.4%)	45 (32.4%)	74 (53.1%)
Chaplains	61	1 (1.6%)	0 (0%)	1 (1.6%)	15 (24.7%)	44 (72.1%)
Pastoral team	61	2 (3.2%)	4 (6.5%)	10 (16.5%)	24 (39.4%)	21 (34.4%)
Admin	6	0 (0%)	0 (0%)	1 (16.7%)	3 (50%)	2 (33.3%)
Weekend	11	0 (0%)	0 (0%)	1 (9.1%)	3 (27.3%)	7 (63.6%)

Table 12.1 is heavily loaded towards the 'successful' end of the spectrum, with 53.1 per cent of the combined results resting there; however, there are variations within the overall base population. Chaplains regarded an overwhelming 72.1 per cent of their encounters to be successful, but this fell to 34.4 per cent with the pastoral team, whose assessments were spread far more evenly across the top three grades.

These figures expose a deficiency in the recording already referred to: what was deemed to constitute 'success'? What aspects of success were missing from 'mostly successful' encounters? Did this assessment result from a potentially successful encounter, which required a return visit to complete the process? The broadness of this descriptor, without further investigation, opens these results to accusations of over-optimism. In particular, the low figures for entirely unsuccessful encounters demanded prompt explanation: it frequently denoted a straight refusal to be visited, or a complete absence of rapport being established with the patient.

Question 16: Who initiated the encounter?

Q16 was included to investigate the claim that perceived demand for the services of chaplaincy is self-generated: were there no chaplains, then there would be no demand.

Table 12.2 Encounter initiators results

Q16: Who initiated the encounter?	Combined count (N = 140)	Chaplains (N = 60)	Pastoral team (N = 61)	Admin (N = 8)	Weekend (N = 11)
Yourself	90 (64.3%)	31 (51.7%)	55 (90.2%)	1 (12.5%)	3 (27.3%)
The other person/s	37 (26.4%)	25 (41.6%)	3 (4.9%)	7 (87.5%)	2 (18.2%)
Mutual	13 (9.3%)	4 (6.7%)	3 (4.9%)	0 (0%)	6 (54.5%)

Chaplains' and pastoral team's figures are widely different: the pastoral team, general visiting in a ward, take the initiative in encountering patients, respecting doubt or refusal. Chaplains tend to be responding to referral requests, hence the lower figure.

Success rates against optimism assessments

As indicated above, the core members of the chaplaincy team met to allocate optimism ratings to members of the pastoral team: there was a high degree of agreement on this matter, which naturally was somewhat delicate. The bulk of chaplains were assessed as 'fairly optimistic'; however, the pastoral team included more members assessed as 'very optimistic', in the sense that pastoral encounters were reviewed in the light of personal salvation, and rapport alone perhaps interpreted as success. Pessimists were rare, and the reluctance to be declared neutral was intriguing. How then did inherent optimism skew members' assessments of the success of their encounters?

Table 12.3 Success assessments set against the 'Optimism Factor'

Optimism / Success	Very pessimistic (N = 0)	Fairly pessimistic (N = 2)	Neutral (N = 13)	Fairly optimistic (N = 100)	Very optimistic (N = 17)
No reply	0	0	1 (7.7%)	1 (1.0%)	0
Unsuccessful	0	0	0	2 (2.0%)	1 (5.9%)
A little successful	0	1 (50%)	2 (15.4%)	1 (1.0%)	0
Partly successful	0	1 (50%)	2 (15.4%)	8 (8.0%)	1(5.9%)
Mostly successful	0	0	5 (38.5%)	30 (30.0%)	7 (41.2%)
Successful encounter	0	0	3 (23.0%)	58 (58.0%)	8 (47.0%)

Though the loading tends to increase towards the bottom and right of the table, even the very optimistic do not claim total success, but are evenly divided between the two top grades: the unsuccessful encounters are reported by the optimists, not the pessimists; pessimism and neutrality are principally represented by assessments of partial or little success.

The typical respondent is fairly optimistic in this system, and 88 per cent of their encounters are in the top two success grades. Even the very optimistic were split quite evenly between mostly and simply successful assessments, so they cannot be easily accused of self-blindness. Given more time interviews could be set up one-to-one with team members, on the subject of these figures. As a side-issue to the project this would be a useful in-house debate.

Success rates compared with complexity

Perhaps success can be confused with achieving personal rapport with a patient, rather than genuinely supporting them; with the significance of sheer length of time spent in their presence being misunderstood? Another enquiry examined this possibility: Table 12.4 examines the relationship between perceived success and complexity of the encounter.

Table 12.4 Success assessments set against complexity of encounters

Success Complexity	No reply	Unsuccessful encounter (N = 3)	A little successful (N = 4)	Partly successful (N = 13)	Mostly successful (N = 45)	Successful encounter (N = 74)
No reply	2					
Simple (N = 18)		2	1	0	4	11
Less simple (N = 17)		0	3	2	9	3
Several topics (N = 43)		0	0	4	20	19
Quite complex (N = 40)		1	0	7	11	21
Complex (N = 21)		0	0	0	1	20

Of the 21 complex encounters reported, 20 were construed as successful; however, of the 40 quite complex encounters the successful rating was only claimed for half. It would appear that there is some justification for suspicion about total success in complex encounters, though below that level the results were mixed, and were perhaps were more credible. Once again, a closer-focused study, perhaps on the encounters of a single chaplain, might pin this elusive definition down; as would patient, staff or carer feedback.

General observations

The survey revealed an active and thoughtful cohort of visitors, both clergy and lay, confronting complex and challenging spiritual situations. The spectrum of subject matter covered is broad and deep, with a realistic assessment of the varying levels of profundity (or lack of it) encountered. Whether encounter content or visiting techniques are being considered, the prosecution of the project itself stimulated enquiry and reflection, an overall spirit of questioning.

There must remain concerns about the recording of levels of perceived success. However, assessments do not appear to have been skewed disproportionately by personal perspective, and the pastoral teams in particular are ready to concede the occasional imperfection. The stage was set for closer examination of departmental and personal aims and objectives

Longer visits appear to be more fruitful than short (ten minutes) visits, but achieving these is a matter of size of team: many patients tire easily, and ten minutes is an appropriate limit for many. Each patient is unique, and the potential for enlargement of the visiting cohort is problematical: the sensible limit of visiting activity may in fact have been reached. Better use of time may be the way ahead.

Having drafted the survey document once, drafting fresh enquiries will be far less laborious; however, data entry is repetitive and time-consuming, so full surveys of this type will need to be restricted to major enquiries. Nevertheless, individual small-scale enquiries could be carried out without computer analysis, making the whole process far less onerous.

Limitations

Existing work pressures, particularly on individual trust chaplains, made recorded encounters variable in quantity and quality; the sample is not therefore a statistically accurate representation of the total number of encounters, though that was invited from all participants. Nor, therefore, does it give an absolute measure of the comparative numbers of encounters with different kinds of team members. The logical requirement of this is to conduct a complete audit of a day's encounters, by a limited number of respondents, though this might prove very onerous to complete from a record-keeping perspective. What are reasonably represented here are the relative levels, across different kinds of team member, of types of encounter; and the different perceptions of team members, and their relative quantification. These findings in themselves represent significant data, although they could, without doubt, be built on in the ways envisaged here.

The future: Implications for further use of the method

This survey has explored the use of a quantitative recording document for capturing both quantitative and qualitative data, and has produced usefully discriminating and detailed data. However, moving down beneath this detailed material, unravelling the motivations, emotions and underlying traumas that may exist in such encounters would require a greater degree of finely observed recording than is possible using such a document. One way forward, already alluded to, would be to seek patient feedback (and indeed staff or relative feedback if such encounters were to be included in a future study). An approach to this might feature initial exploratory interviews, designed to establish an in-depth picture of patient perspectives, followed by standardised interviews or questionnaires developed from that picture, and designed to produce comparative, statistically significant data (see Oppenheim 1992, Chapter 5). The method discussed in this chapter is perfectly capable of being extended to staff and to family members, or focused down to a particular group or even an individual.

To summarise, the weakness of the approach discussed in this chapter, in comparison with the aims of the MDS (South Yorkshire Workforce Development Confederation 2004), is the incomplete quantification of data relating to encounters that resulted from the decision not to ask team members to record every encounter. This decision, as indicated, could be reversed in future studies; at which point the data generated would be a more nuanced quantification than that envisaged for an MDS. Where this study extends beyond the aims of establishing an MDS, is in the investigation of the nature of the encounters. The research discussed here begins to explore and quantify the different kinds of encounter with patients that different types of chaplaincy team member are engaged in. Further, it begins to explore team members' perceptions of the nature of those encounters, in terms of whether they are, *inter alia*, mundane or spiritual, more or less complex and more or less successful. As noted, this exploration relies too much on the subjective judgement of the team members in this study. But future research, suggested above, that correlated chaplaincy and patient/staff/relative perspectives would give greater depth to the approach; and allow for quantitative testing designed to establish representative views.

Generating an atmosphere of self-enquiry was stimulating and invigorating, developing the chaplaincy team's spirit of enquiry, and contributing to their developing reflective practice. Although the project may have generated as many questions as answers, the questions arising, discussed above, are deeper and more important than the originals. Seen as a pilot project, the research considered in this chapter makes a small, but significant contribution to healthcare chaplaincy becoming more able to demonstrate an evidence base that establishes good practice (and stimulates reflection on its development); and justifies the use of public money to resource spiritual care.

REFERENCES

Armstrong, K. (2000) *The Battle for God.* London: Harper Collins.

Barkham, M., Stiles, W.B., Lambert, K.J. and Mellor-Clark, J. (2010) 'Building a Rigorous and Relevant Knowledge Base for the Psychological Therapies.' In M. Barkham, G.E. Hardy and J. Mellor-Clark (eds) *Developing and Delivering Practice-Based Evidence: A Guide for the Psychological Therapies: Effectiveness Research in Counselling and the Psychological Therapies.* Chichester, UK: Wiley and Sons.

Baxendale, R.D. (2010) 'What initial insights into the efficacy of the spiritual care offered by the Department of Pastoral and Spiritual Care, Plymouth Hospitals NHS Trust, can be identified by an ethnographic survey of a week's activity of the Department?' Unpublished MTh dissertation, Cardiff University.

BBC (2009) 'Trust defends "spiritual" policy.' BBC News, 5 March. Available at: http://news.bbc.co.uk/1/hi/england/hampshire/7926724.stm (accessed 20 February 2015).

BBC (2013) 'Chaplaincy services cut in 40% of English NHS hospital trusts.' BBC News, 27 June. Available at: www.bbc.co.uk/news/uk-england-23011620 (accessed 20 February 2015).

Bevan, E.G., Chee, L.C., McGhee, S.M. and McInnes, G.T. (1993) 'Patients' attitudes to participation in clinical trials.' *British Journal of Clinical Pharmacology 35,* 2, 204–207.

BHA (2014) 'Non-religious beliefs.' British Humanist Association. Available at: https://humanism.org.uk/humanism/humanism-today/non-religious-beliefs/ (accessed 20 February 2015).

Bower, P. and Gilbody, S. (2010) 'The Current View of Evidence and Evidence-based Practice.' In M. Barkham, G.E. Hardy and J. Mellor-Clark (eds) *Developing and Delivering Practice-Based Evidence: A Guide for the Psychological Therapies: Effectiveness Research in Counselling and the Psychological Therapies.* Chichester, UK: Wiley and Sons.

Brierley, P. (2000) 'The Tide is Running Out.' In S. Bruce (2002) *God is Dead. Secularization in the West.* Oxford: Blackwell.

Brierley, P (2006) *Pulling out of the Nosedive: A Contemporary Picture of Churchgoing – What the 2005 English Church Census Reveals.* London: Christian Research.

Brown, N. (1999) 'A chaplaincy fetter from America.' *Scottish Journal of Healthcare Chaplaincy 2,* 1, 15–19.

Bruce, S. (2003) 'The Demise of Christianity in Britain.' In G. Davie, P. Heelas and L. Woodhead (eds.) *Predicting Religion: Christian, Secular and Alternative Futures.* Aldershot, UK: Ashgate.

Bunniss, S., Mowat, H. and Snowden, A. (2013) 'Community chaplaincy listening: Practical theology in action.' *Scottish Journal of Healthcare Chaplaincy 16,* 42–51.

Carr-Hill, R. (1995) 'Welcome? To the brave new world of evidence based medicine.' *Social Science and Medicine 41,* 11, 1467–1468.

Charmaz, K. (2000) 'Grounded Theory: Objectivist and Constructivist Methods.' In N.K. Denzin and Y.S. Lincoln (eds) *Handbook of Qualitative Research* (second edition). Thousand Oaks, CA: Sage.

Charmaz, K. (2006) *Constructing Grounded Theory: A Practical Guide through Qualitative Analysis.* London: Sage.

Christian, R. (2011) *Costing the heavens: Chaplaincy services in English NHS provider Trusts 2009/10.* Available at: www.secularism.org.uk/uploads/nss-chaplaincy-report-2011.pdf (accessed 20 February 2015). London: National Secular Society.

Cobb, M. (2008) 'Growing research in the practice of chaplains.' *The Journal of Health Care Chaplaincy 9*, 1/2, 4–9.

Cooper, R.S. (2011) 'Case study of a chaplain's spiritual care for a patient with advanced metastatic breast cancer.' *Journal of Health Care Chaplaincy 17*, 1, 19–37.

Corbin, J. and Strauss, A. (2008) *Basics of Qualitative Research* (third edition). Thousand Oaks, CA: Sage.

Corrington, R.S. (1998) 'Empirical Theology and its Divergence from Process Thought.' In R.A. Badham (ed.) *Introduction to Christian Theology: Contemporary North American Perspectives.* Louisville, KN: Westminster John Knox.

Davie, G. (2002) *Europe: The Exceptional Case. Parameters of Faith in the Modern World.* London: Darton, Longman and Todd.

Davies, M. (2013) 'Hospital chaplaincy under the knife, study finds.' *Church Times*, 28 June. Available at: www.churchtimes.co.uk/articles/2013/28-june/news/uk/hospital-chaplaincy-under-the-knife,-study-finds (accessed 20 February 2015).

Denzin, N.K. and Lincoln, Y.S. (2000) 'The Discipline and Practice of Qualitative Research.' In N.K. Denzin and Y.S. Lincoln (eds) *Handbook of Qualitative Research* (second edition). Thousand Oaks, CA: Sage.

Faulkner, A. (2004) *The Ethics of Survivor Research: Guidelines for the Ethical Conduct of Research Carried Out by Mental Health Service Users and Survivors.* Bristol, UK: Policy Press.

Faulkner, A. (2012) 'Participation and Service User Involvement.' In D. Harper and A. Thompson (eds) *Qualitative Research Methods in Health and Psychotherapy.* Chichester, UK: Wiley.

Fitchett, G. (2011) 'Making our case(s).' *Journal of Health Care Chaplaincy 17*, 1, 3–18.

Fitchett, G. and Grossoehme, D. (2012) 'Healthcare Chaplaincy as a Research-informed Profession.' In S.B. Roberts (2012) *Professional Spiritual and Pastoral Care: A Practical Clergy and Chaplain's Handbook.* Woodstock, VT: SkyLight Paths.

Fitchett, G. and Nolan, S. (2015) *Spiritual Care in Practice: Case Studies in Healthcare Chaplaincy.* London: Jessica Kingsley Publishers.

Foskett, J. (2013) 'Is there evidence-based confirmation of the value of pastoral and spiritual care? An invitation to a conversation.' *Health and Social Care Chaplaincy 1*, 1, 83–90.

Francis, L.J., Robbins, M. and Astley, J. (eds) (2009) *Empirical Theology in Texts and Tables: Qualitative, Quantitative and Comparative Perspectives.* Leiden, the Netherlands: Brill.

Francis, R. (2013) 'Report of the Mid Staffordshire NHS Foundation Trust public inquiry: executive summary.' London: HMSO.

Goodhead, A. (2008) 'The importance of the nursing role in spiritual care of patients.' *End of Life Care 2*, 2, 34–37.

Handzo, G.F., Cobb, M., Holmes, C., Kelly, E. and Sinclair, S. (2014) 'Outcomes for professional health care chaplaincy: An international call to action.' *Journal of Health Care Chaplaincy 20*, 2, 43–53.

Heelas, P. and Woodhead, L. (2005) *The Spiritual Revolution: Why Religion is Giving Way to Spirituality.* Oxford: Blackwell.

HMSO (2005) 'Mental Capacity Act.' London: The Stationery Office.

Hundley, V. (1999) 'Evidence based practice: What is it? And why does it matter?' *Scottish Journal of Healthcare Chaplaincy 2*, 1, 11–14.

Jamieson, A. (2002) *A Churchless Faith: Faith Journeys Beyond the Churches.* London. SPCK.

Jamieson, A., McIntosh, J. and Thompson, A. (2006) *Church Leavers: Faith Journeys Five Years On.* London: SPCK.

Kendall, T., Glover, N., Taylor, C. and Pilling, S. (2011) 'Quality, bias and service user experience in healthcare: 10 years of mental health guidelines at the UK National Collaborating Centre for Mental Health.' *International Review of Psychiatry 23*, 4, 342–351.

King, M., Jones, L., Barnes, K., Low, J., Walker, C., Wilkinson, S., Mason, C., Sutherland, J. and Tookman, A. (2006) 'Measuring spiritual belief: Development and standardization of a beliefs and values scale.' *Psychological Medicine 36*, 3, 417–425.

King, S.D.W. (2012) 'Facing fears and counting blessings: A case study of a chaplain's faithful companioning a cancer patient.' *Journal of Health Care Chaplaincy 18*, 1–2, 3–22.

Lassiter, L.E. (2005) *The Chicago Guide to Collaborative Ethnography*. Chicago, IL: University of Chicago Press.

MacKinnon, K. (2012) 'What light do the beliefs of volunteers in University Hospital Southampton NHS Foundation Trust cast on the secularity of the contemporary NHS and what are the implications for chaplaincy?' Unpublished MTh dissertation, Cardiff University.

McCurdy, D. and Fitchett, G. (2011) 'Ethical issues in case study publication: "Making our case(s)" ethically.' *Journal of Health Care Chaplaincy 17*, 1, 55–74.

McSherry, E. (1987) 'The need and appropriateness of measurement and research in chaplaincy: Its criticalness for patient care and chaplain department survival post 1987.' *Journal of Health Care Chaplaincy 1*, 1, 3–42.

McSherry, W. (2007) *The Meaning of Spirituality and Spiritual Care within Nursing and Health Care Practice.* London: MA Healthcare.

McSherry, W. (2011) 'RCN spirituality survey 2010: A report by the Royal College of Nursing on members' views on spirituality and spiritual care in nursing practice.' Royal College of Nursing: London.

Mann, H. (1853) 'Census of Great Britain, 1851, Religious worship (England and Wales): Report and Tables.' London: Eyre and Spottiswoode. Available at: www.histpop.org/ohpr/servlet/AssociatedPageBrowser?path=Browse&active=yes&mno=32&tocstate=expandnew&display=sections&display=tables&display=pagetitles&pageseq=1&assoctitle=The%20religious%20worship%20census%20of%201851&assocpagelabel= (accessed 20 February 2015).

Mowat, H. (2008) 'The potential for efficacy of healthcare chaplaincy and spiritual care provision in the NHS (UK): A scoping review of recent research.' Aberdeen, UK: Mowat Research Limited.

Mowat, H. and Swinton, J. (2007) *What do chaplains do? The role of the chaplain in meeting the spiritual needs of patients* (2nd edition). Aberdeen: Mowat Research Limited.

Mowat, H., Bunniss, S. and Kelly, E. (2012) 'Community chaplaincy listening: Working with general practitioners to support patient wellbeing.' *Scottish Journal of Healthcare Chaplaincy 15*, 1, 21–26.

Nicholls, V. (ed.) (2002) 'Taken seriously: The Somerset spirituality project.' London: The Mental Health Foundation.

NIHR (2013) 'Good practice guidance for involving people with experience of mental health problems in research.' Available at: www.rds-sw.nihr.ac.uk/documents/NIHR_MHRN_Involving_Mental_Health_Problems_Research2013.pdf (accessed 20 February 2015).

Nolan, S. (2011) 'The importance of critical thinking in evidence-based practice.' *PlainViews 8*, 22. Available at: www.plainviews.org (accessed 20 February 2015).

Nolan, S. and Holloway, M. (2014) *A–Z of Spirituality*. Basingstoke, UK: Palgrave Macmillan.

NSS (2011) 'New study of chaplains shows little benefit to clinical outcomes.' National Secular Society. Available at: www.secularism.org.uk/new-study-of-chaplains-shows-lit.html (accessed 20 February 2015).

ONS (2012) 'Religion in England and Wales 2011.' Office for National Statistics. Available at: www.ons.gov.uk/ons/rel/census/2011-census/key-statistics-for-local-authorities-in-england-and-wales/rpt-religion.html (accessed 20 February 2015).

Oppenheim, A.N. (1992) *Questionnaire Design, Interviewing and Attitude Measurement.* London: Bloomsbury Publishing.

Paley, J. (2009) 'Keep the NHS secular.' *Nursing Standard 23*, 43, 26–27.

Puchalski, C.M. and Ferrell, B. (2010) *Making Health Care Whole: Integrating Spirituality into Patient Care.* West Conshohocken, PA: Templeton Press.

Raffay, J. (2012) 'Are our mental health practices beyond HOPE?' *Journal of Health Care Chaplaincy, 12*, 2, 68–80.

Raffay, J. (2013) 'How staff and patient experience shapes our perception of spiritual care in a psychiatric setting.' *Journal of Nursing Management 22*, 940–950.

Reed, P.G. (1992) 'An emerging paradigm for the investigation of spirituality in nursing.' *Research in Nursing and Health 15*, 5, 349–357.

Risk, J.L. (2013) 'Building a new life: A chaplain's theory based case study of chronic illness.' *Journal of Health Care Chaplaincy 19*, 81–98.

Sackett, D.L., Rosenberg, W.M.C., Gray, J.A.M., Haynes, R.B. and Richardson, W.S. (1996) 'Evidence based medicine: What it is and what it isn't.' *British Medical Journal International Edition 312.7023,* 71. Available at: search.proquest.com/docview/203965522?account id=48280 (accessed 20 February 2015).

Snowden, A., Telfer, I., Kelly, E., Bunniss, S. and Mowat, H. (2013a) 'The construction of the Lothian PROM.' *Scottish Journal of Healthcare Chaplaincy 16*, 3–12.

Snowden, A., Telfer, I., Kelly, E., Bunniss, S. and Mowat, H. (2013b) '"I was able to talk about what was on my mind": The operationalisation of person centred care.' *Scottish Journal of Healthcare Chaplaincy 16*, 13–22.

South Yorkshire Workforce Development Confederation (2003) 'Caring for the spirit: A strategy for the chaplaincy and spiritual healthcare workforce.' London: South Yorkshire Workforce Development Confederation.

South Yorkshire Workforce Development Confederation (2004) 'Consultative proposals for a minimum data set for spiritual healthcare. Caring for the spirit: Implementation plan. Guidance Note 5.' London: South Yorkshire Workforce Development Confederation.

Speck, P.W. (2005) 'A standard for research in health care chaplaincy.' *The Journal of Health Care Chaplaincy 6*, 1, 26–40.

Sweeney, A., Beresford, P., Faulkner, A., Nettle, M. and Rose, D (eds) (2009) *This is Survivor Research.* Ross-on-Wye, UK: PCCS Books.

Swift, C. (2009) *Hospital Chaplaincy in the Twenty-first Century: The Crisis of Spiritual Care on the NHS.* Farnham, UK and Burlington, VA: Ashgate.

Swinton, J. (1999) 'Editorial.' *Scottish Journal of Healthcare Chaplaincy 2*, 1, 1–2.

Taylor, C. (2007) *A Secular Age.* Cambridge, MA: Belknap Press of Harvard University Press.

Terry, W., Olson, L.G., Ravenscroft, P., Wilss, L. and Boulton-Lewis, G. (2006) 'Hospice patients' views on research in palliative care.' *International Medicine Journal 36*, 406–413.

van der Ven, J.A. (1998) *Practical Theology: An Empirical Approach.* Leuven, the Netherlands: Peeters.

Wampold, B.E. (2010) 'Foreword.' In M. Barkham, G.E. Hardy and J. Mellor-Clark (eds) *Developing and Delivering Practice-Based Evidence: A Guide for the Psychological Therapies: Effectiveness Research in Counselling and the Psychological Therapies.* Chichester, UK: Wiley and Sons.

Warner, R. (2010) *Secularization and its Discontents.* London: Continuum.

Weber, M., Gerth, H.H. and Wright Mills, C. (1948) *From Max Weber: Essays in Sociology.* New York: Routledge.

PART 4

Critical Issues in Spiritual Care

CHAPTER 13

The Practice of Spiritual Care in the Context of Suffering

Questions for the Self as a 'Spiritual Being'

Peter Sedgwick

Introduction

The argument of this chapter begins with the work of the philosopher Charles Taylor, who has offered a well-received account of the subjectivity of the modern self (Taylor 2007). This is followed by a brief description of the way the concept of spirituality is treated in modern writing about chaplaincy, mental illness and dying. The particular interest of this chapter is the strength of a person's spirituality in the face of great suffering, whether caused by factors that may be psychological, physical or social (such as genocide, or trauma in war), or even a combination of all three. The chapter poses three questions to the healthcare chaplains who write in this section of the volume. First, how does such suffering affect the delivery of spiritual care by chaplains? Second, what is the nature of this spiritual care, in the face of suffering? As a Christian theologian I wish to echo Clayton in Chapter 16. Jesus Christ is the source of wholeness hidden in the practice of spiritual care. Issues of supersessionism (the replacement of Judaism as the chosen or covenant people by Christianity) are also discussed, so that what may be called the 'making present of Christ' does not become a monolithic or oppressive practice. Third, how does the chaplain embody Christ in this making present, or their performance of spiritual care? Finally I offer some reflections on the nature of Christ's presence in suffering and death, as mediated by the chaplains who have written in this section of the book.

Taylor's argument

Like most contemporary philosophers, sociologists and historians, Taylor no longer believes that one can begin any modern understanding of what it means to be a person by arguing that the person can be defined in religious terms. Religion here is defined as the activity of an institutional body, such as Christianity, or denominations that collectively make up the body which is Christianity. Denominations are, for instance, Methodism or the Anglican Church. For an example of such turning away from the significance of religion, David Reynolds' *The Long Shadow* (Reynolds 2013) is a good example. Reynolds is Professor of International History at Cambridge University and has written a magisterial and well-reviewed book on the impact of the First World War on the 20th century. Although it is impossible to exclude Christianity from its 600 pages, nowhere is the interplay of the war and religious belief and practice ever attempted. It is simply excluded. Reynolds would be typical of many in seeing the practice of religion as belonging to a past era for the majority of European people and no longer of significance for most intellectuals. It is, of course, possible to argue with this thesis, and many have, but I mention it because it frames and contextualises Taylor's approach.

Taylor is himself a practising Roman Catholic, who is a highly regarded philosopher, especially on Hegel. Taylor (2007) sets out a conceptual framework for understanding subjectivity, which has been widely accepted. To understand the person, one must see the concepts of 'self' and 'person' as closely related categories. The modern self is seen as essentially autonomous, self-directed and expressive. The neo-Durkheimian age (roughly the 19th and first part of the 20th centuries) was one where nation states used theistic religion, and then created forms of nationalism-as-religion to bind their citizens into a cohesion that enabled national self-consciousness to be achieved. This age is now drawing to its close, and the traumas of the 1960s, especially in the USA, France and Germany in the epic year of 1968, mean that religion is no longer to be seen as an agent of social cohesion, as Durkheim had argued (Durkheim 1912/2008; Lash 1996; Martin 1980). What has taken its place is an emphasis on the person as a being who can enter into carefully circumscribed relationships. Such a person has at her heart a self that is, as we shall see below, equally carefully defined. The self must be nurtured, and this leads to a demand for authenticity and an acceptance of spiritual pluralism (Taylor 2007, p.490). Taylor believes that the modern self can, and should, enter into relationship with transcendence. Taylor ultimately identifies transcendence with God. However, he doubts whether most people today find their relationship with God via a close identification with the churches. Their ancestors once belonged to particular denominations, but they no longer do so. In this sense, Taylor speaks, in a slightly exaggerated manner, of the end of religion in Europe and North America. More especially, Taylor argues for the end (empirically, but also normatively) of religion as an institutional identity that collectively gives social cohesion to the nation state, or the inhabitants of a city, as Catholicism, Methodism or Anglicanism certainly did throughout the 19th and early 20th century. This is the Durkheimian age, and it is over. All that we have in post-modern Europe and North America is what Taylor calls ever more fragmented 'spiritual pluralism'. Institutional religion is now in its demise for Taylor, and it will not revive its former social dominance.

Chaplaincy has responded to this cultural change with enormous changes in its practice, and it maintains a constant dialogue with patients and staff in health care (Swift 2009). So the autonomous self, and the culture of which the self is but a part, develops a discourse that can be called 'spiritual', and this discourse has to be constructed within clinical care settings, negotiated in the public square and researched. That is the burden of this volume so far. Could a patient or a staff member in clinical care be seen, then, not as religious *per se*, but as a spiritual person, who could be ministered to by chaplaincy? The answer is a series of conditional replies, or affirmations. Yes, if it is given that the construction and negotiation of the existence of spiritual discourse and practice within clinical care is successful. Yes, the patient or staff member can be seen as spiritual given a willingness (at least in part) for the patient (or staff member) to participate in the cultural, social and personal practices that constitute 'being spiritual'. Then, and only then, the patient/staff member qua autonomous self is duly redefined, and understood as a patient/staff member qua spiritual self. Who would understand them in this way? Certainly chaplains could, and do so. Equally, the patient or staff member can be seen in this way by theologians, perhaps by sociologists, ethnographers and clinicians, and even perhaps by themselves. In so doing the self enters into spiritual relationships, and so gives up some of its own autonomy.

Taylor describes the modern self as buffered:

All thought, feeling and purpose, all the features we normally can ascribe to agents, must be in minds which are distinct from the 'outer' world. The buffered self begins to find the ideas of spirits, moral forces, causal powers with a purposive bent, close to incomprehensible. (Taylor 2007, p.539)

There is not only an inner/outer distinction between mind and world; there is also what Taylor calls 'a rich vocabulary of interiority, an inner realm of thought and feeling to be explored' (Taylor 2007, p.539). This interiority is based on disciplines of self-examination, the rise of Romanticism, the ethic of authenticity and the belief in the self having inner depths. Once there was a belief in evil spirits; now we think of mental illness. Once we saw the world as enchanted and having a rich symbolism; now, after the rise in our culture of the discipline of psychoanalysis, we locate this symbolism in the psyche. There are close links with the discipline of self-control, zones of intimacy within which we share our depths of feeling and affinity and an awareness of our individuality. In all of this, the commitment to self-responsibility, the establishment of new social order through an instrumental stance towards the world and time, and the end of ideas of cosmic order, means that the world is seen as immanent. The rise of natural science after Galileo dovetails perfectly with this understanding of the self. Taylor shows how many thinkers reject religion as emanating 'from a childish lack of courage. We need to…face reality' (Taylor 2007, p.561). Taylor denies, however, that a rejection of religion need lead to a denial of a relationship with God.

Indeed, as Taylor says, the contemporary world has seen many attempts to create a spirituality that does not reject all that has been said above, and still finds a place for a non-material reality. Taylor juxtaposes a therapeutic and a spiritual understanding of the self as it deals with what were once called the fruits of sin, such as impotence, emptiness, anguish and incapacity. Therapy sees these conditions as a sickness, or as a pathology, and may treat them by behavioural means, or by drugs, or by psychoanalysis. These conditions are to be removed by delving into 'the unavoidable, deep psychic conflicts in our make-up' (Taylor 2007, p.621), but for the secular therapist the analysis has no moral lesson for us.

We strive to understand them in order to reduce their force, to become able to live with them. On the crucial issue, what we have morally or spiritually to learn from our suffering, it is firmly on the therapeutic side: the answer is nothing. (Taylor 2007, p.621)

The alternative (Taylor's own one) is a spiritual perspective. It argues that we are drawn to live in relation to what can be defined as spiritual reality. Unease, anguish and emptiness are not only symptomatic of inner conflict, as a therapist would say, but they are also perceptions of a lack or misdirection in our lives. They reveal that we are failing to engage fully with our truest good, or a more real self. 'The goal must be to find a more adequate response to the spiritual reality, not to flee from it' (Taylor 2007, p.622). The answer still lies in the restoration of a relationship with God.

Spirituality in healthcare

There has been a great deal of writing about the replacement of religion by spirituality in the past few decades, and what that might mean for someone in medical care. Such writers as Cobb and Robshaw (1998), Gilbert (2011), Swift (2009), Swinton (2001) and Swinton and Payne (2009) have all pointed to the centrality of spirituality in the practice of healthcare chaplaincy. Just as Taylor does, Swinton resists translating spirituality into psychological terms (Swinton 2001). These desires refer to dimensions that include, but also transcend, psychological explanation. Swinton defends this transcendental element from 'a deep, intuitive sense of affirmation' (Swinton 2001, p.25), which gives him a sense of intuitive knowledge. The central features of spirituality include meaning (making sense of life); value (beliefs and standards that relate to the truth, beauty and worth of a thought, object or behaviour); transcendence, which he defines as beyond self, thus enabling him to include non-theistic dimensions; connections with others, the environment and God or ultimate reality; and finally, becoming. All these are congruent with the argument offered by Taylor in the preceding paragraphs.

Among the many questions to be put to this argument is the one that asks 'how strong or resilient is this spiritual self?' (Other questions, not pursued here, include the relationship of the autonomous self and the spiritual self: do they overlap, interpenetrate, remain distinct entities in different cultural contexts, or how is the relationship to be described? However, those questions are for the earlier part of this volume.) Suffering is my preferred term, but it could also be described as a 'limit condition'. Computer manuals refer to 'limit conditions', which create stress (the immediate symptoms of malfunction, such as an operating system losing data, or even crashing), and the degradation of performance of the operating system (the long-term malfunction). Analogously, human life can also encounter limit conditions, which are indicated initially by signs of severe stress, such as extreme emotion, irrational behaviour and breakdown in relationships. These also create the long-term degradation of the very possibilities of human life. However, suffering is a more direct and immediate expression of this reality.

It is a constant theme of contemporary clinical care that great suffering, which can test and break a person's belief in the goodness of life, and the value of their own existence, includes enduring physical and mental realities. These include continuing psychopathic disorder, sometimes allied with irresolvable guilt at past crimes; long-term mental illness (including dementia and Mild Cognitive Impairment); and the awareness of terminal illness, especially among children. There is also, of course, long-term physical degradation, and progressive (and terminal) illness, but these issues are not touched upon in this section of the volume.

Swinton relates spirituality to meaninglessness and depression, thus offering an answer to the question posed above about the strength of spirituality and religious faith in the face of suffering. Swinton notes that not only is meaning sucked out of life through depression, but it also drains the psychological strength to fight it (Swinton 2001, p.117). What is redemptive are understanding and empathy, which become in themselves forms of spiritual experience. Another source of hope is liturgy and worship, where the non-cognitive elements of ritual and symbol become important (Swinton 2001, pp.128–129). Scripture ceases to be propositional, in a way that affirms truths propositionally, which are then applied to one's life. Rather, the act of identifying with figures or types encountered in scripture becomes redemptive: 'This person in scripture could be/becomes me...' The existential crisis in the Psalmist is placed within the community of faith, which holds the text as its path to God in a way that cannot be understood, but can be trusted as a 'rite of passage' through darkness to trust. However, the community of faith is also, for Swinton, not to be equated too easily with institutional religion. There is both overlap between the two concepts and separation.

Healthcare chaplaincy and spirituality

A crucial question then becomes the validity of the practice of spirituality when faced with such suffering. There are three aspects to this question, which press hard on the particular three chaplains (Wharton, Thody and Clayton) who write in this section. First, in what ways do patients' sufferings, which chaplains themselves experience, affect their delivery of spiritual care? More precisely, if one is a chaplain dealing with enduring mental illness, the onset of Mild Cognitive Impairment, or child mortality, how do you continue to engage spiritually? Second, what is the nature of this spiritual care, or what I will go on to call the 'making present of Christ'? Third, how does the chaplain embody Christ in this making present, or their performance of spiritual care? The rest of this chapter will look at how the three chaplains mentioned respond to these three questions. At the end there is also a reflection on the nature of the presence of Christ. Christ's reality in the complexity of human relationships always fashions new questions for the self and the possibility of a relationship with him.

The delivery of spiritual care

Let me turn to the first of these aspects, which is the interaction of spirituality and the facing of suffering. Long-term mental illness is the subject of Thody's chapter (Chapter 14). He analyses the response of a fictional patient, in a high secure forensic setting, who has unresolved torment from the harm caused to others by her past crimes, and the ongoing reality of her 'incurable' (however defined) mental illness. Thody discusses what the most appropriate response would be by this person, and concludes that assisted suicide can sometimes be the most appropriate form of spirituality. This powerful contribution is also echoed by Newell (2002), who was governor of Grendon Prison, which was both a high security prison and a therapeutic establishment. Newell, who is a member of the Society of Friends, saw assisted suicide as a response to the reality of the possibility of life imprisonment without release, and his chapter in a volume on the future of the criminal justice system describes how he gave permission for this to happen when he was governor:

> Through therapy Gary came to an understanding of the effects his actions on others' life...he began his fast that concluded with his death three and a half months later. He made his peace with his family and all who had dealings

with him in prison. He expressed forgiveness for all of us – he did not want any of us to feel guilty or angry about his death. We should accept his death as a triumph over the past. Although a desperately sad time for many of us, there was a haunting dignity and humanity about Gary that will stay with me for all of my life. (Newell 2002, pp.148–149)

A different limit condition within clinical care today is that of dementia. This is discussed by Wharton (Chapter 15), in relationship to Mild Cognitive Impairment. Wharton uses an ethnographic piece of qualitative research, which he undertook among patients living at home, but receiving care from a mental NHS trust. The need for clinical judgement emphasises in Wharton's view the need for a multi-disciplinary and multi-dimensional approach to care. He continues:

Effective holistic care of those with mental illness necessitates as much an understanding of their social narrative, spirituality, values and connectedness, as it does of their neuropathology.

Mild Cognitive Impairment is a syndrome which has a significant chance of developing into dementia. Figures vary on the rate of conversion from MCI to dementia, or Alzheimer's disease and related disorders (ADRD). Some say that it is as low as 10% per annum, while others give rates as high as 50%.

ADRD is a complex and cruel disease. The most familiar characteristic is memory loss; but others include language, perception, problem solving, abstract thinking and judgement. Sufferers' inability to tolerate stress of any kind also leads to negative changes in personality and behaviour.

(Rees 2012, p.1)

She notes that 'many clinical staff are uncomfortable when confronted with the spiritual needs of patients' (Rees 2012, p.5). Relationships with those with Mild Cognitive Impairment and Alzheimer's disease and related disorders are enhanced by practices of spirituality. 'Higher levels of private religious activities and of spirituality predict slower cognitive decline in patients with AD' (Rees 2012, p.8). An article by Kaufman *et al.* (2007) notes that it is not levels of attendance at religious services that shows this correlation, because 'this aged, frail, and cognitively impaired group is likely to have greater difficulties in attending religious services, and thus spirituality/religiosity may be better expressed through private religious activities' (Kaufman *et al.* 2007, p.1511).

Finally, Clayton (Chapter 16) reflects on his work over many years as a lay chaplain in a children's hospice, where enduring suffering is created by the progressive incapacity of the children and their awareness of their approaching death, and the agonised response of the parents. There are different aspects of this parental response, sometimes moments of great fear, sometimes frenetic activity, sometimes simply passivity and withdrawal.

As Clayton writes elsewhere, the experience of families in a children's hospice, 'can shake their faith in the foundations of life, and activity can sometimes become restless or frenetic…the profound disconnection of dying…withdrawing, turning to the wall in his hospital bed, and no longer communicating' (Clayton 2013, pp.38, 40).

The nature of spiritual care

So the next question is, 'What is the nature of this spiritual care?' Authenticity and the construction of spiritual care are but the beginnings of recognition of the dynamic interaction of God, human beings and nature. In the Christian tradition this can be called 'a making present of Christ'. The making present of Christ can be in many ways. First, there is Thody's account of being present in a high security forensic psychiatric setting. Thody reflects on the changes in his own spirituality, as he wrestled with the ethical issue of assisted suicide for those in what he calls 'mental torment'. Thody offers a highly ethical account of the spiritual dilemma, but this is interwoven in his chapter (Chapter 14) with the Christian passion narrative, where the dying Christ in awful suffering radiates love and compassion. Christ is accompanied by 'those close to him, his mother and the disciple, who must have longed for him to live, yet also understood the death and stood by him when others ran away'. The possibility, and legalisation of, assisted suicide is an ethical question, but it is also a religious one, where the very manner of the act of dying can give meaning both to the death itself and the preceding life. Christ is an authoritative presence in Thody's narrative, controlling the parameters of the explanatory narrative.

Second, there is what Wharton (Chapter 15) calls 'transformative, sacred narratives of our patients…the potency of storytelling in community and small groups'. He also draws attention to the importance of ritual, both religious and social, whether family or communal. The practice of spirituality in coming to terms with dementia is also studied by psychologists (Kaufman *et al.*, 2007). Wharton uses categories such as resilience, maturity and living with dichotomous experiences. Spiritual growth is an appropriate term to use in spite of cognitive degeneration. Another aspect of spiritual care is the relationship between carer and patient. Rees writes:

> *Thus, valuing a person enables us to discover new facets of their personality. While these may not always be pleasant (e.g., anger and frustration), they present us with a unique opportunity to learn more about the person 'within', and to celebrate things about them that, perhaps without the ADRD would have remained hidden to us. (Rees 2012, p.7)*

Furthermore, Rees goes on, in words that will be echoed by Hardy at the end of this chapter:

> *The biggest myth surrounding worshipping with those with ADRD is that nothing can be done. On the contrary, we must look for new ways of connecting the spirit of the sufferer with God's Spirit. We must hold fast to the promise that though their bodies are failing God inwardly renews them daily (2Cor: 4:16). (Rees 2012, p.12)*

Third, Clayton (Chapter 16) goes into great detail about his experience of symbol and ritual. Among them are symbols of wholeness, contemplation, rituals of healing and blessing. There are many rituals, actions and symbolic objects, such as a colourful coffin, memory trees, nativity plays and of course the ritual of the funeral itself. Creating a symbolic world of spiritual care takes careful attention and much time: it does not just happen. It needs to contain meaning in itself, and speak both to the reality of the child as he or she approaches death; the family's experience; and to the religious tradition which the family holds. For Clayton himself as a chaplain, there is also the necessity of expressing this communication in a way that honours the integrity of Christianity, or in other words being faithful to Christ.

The chaplain and the embodying of spiritual care: Making Christ present

The third question asks how the chaplain embodies this making present of Christ. What is striking, in particular, is Thody's powerful phrase in Chapter 14 about how Jesus' mother and disciple at the crucifixion 'stood by him when others ran away'. This is the role of the chaplain, who, often under great stress, stands by, and understands the death. Thody places himself within the typology of the witnessing, suffering and ultimately loving mother of Jesus, and also of the disciple (one wonders, incidentally, for someone who once described himself as a 'fairly traditional "conservative catholic"', with which of the two he most identifies) as the self-accepted and willed death draws to its close. It is no wonder that Thody speaks of having 'found myself in tension with fellow clergy when the issue of supporting a person's desire to end their life has arisen'. He speaks of having his Anglican spirituality, 'set very much by the established church', deeply challenged by the practice of spiritual care as a chaplain within a forensic psychiatric setting.

Wharton writes his chapter both as a chaplain and as a researcher, seeing himself as an officeholder inside a large and complex organisation, which is a hospital trust in the NHS. Such an officeholder would be someone who develops work-plans to improve the chaplaincy's provision of services. This is a more functional approach, which emphasises consultation with local faith-based groups. The chaplain mediates between local community projects and the delivery of care from the hospital trust. It is important to note that those receiving care were all living in their own home at the time of the research. The chaplain becomes their spiritual resource as they interact at the same time both with their own religious communities and with the hospital.

Clayton emphasises his own contemplative stance. He writes 'Inner stillness is integral to the way in which we bear the cost of the present moment' (Clayton 2013, p.35). The chaplain becomes the focus of the spiritual care that everyone in the hospice gives. He is a living symbol, embodying and personalising a dimension of spiritual care that can be nebulous and unclear. So Clayton directly understands the chaplain as embodying the presence of Christ. In a way that is highly sacramental, but not in and of itself a sacrament, the chaplain becomes like Jesus. He writes:

> the mystery of a child's death can also call a Christian chaplain to grow in and embody wholeness and holiness. Such a death can summon us to respond personally by living a more fully human life… In following the self-emptying of Jesus in the Christian tradition (Phil. 2.7), a contemplative stance can free chaplains from unnecessary activities in order that we might face the emptiness of death with others. (Clayton 2013, pp.41, 44)

Yet the chaplain is not the only symbol of such care. The child as he or she approaches death becomes the means by which God speaks to relatives, carers and staff. Clayton speaks of not theologising this symbol but living it with the mother, metaphorically and literally at the foot of the (symbol of the) cross, following the chaplain in the pain of dereliction as the chaplain also lives out what it means to walk the holy life. The mother accompanies the child and the chaplain walks beside her, in a mutually enriching relationship, the one looking to the other. Beyond them both is the physical space of the chapel, where the funeral will take place.

> *As the baby had been christened in hospital and relatives had lit candles for her in our chapel, I asked the parents if they would like to pray for her there. To my surprise, the whole family gathered with the little baby. They spent the time not only saying some prayers but also sharing together their thankfulness for her, their profound grief, and their love and affection for one another. My invitation to pray in the chapel created a different physical and emotional space for them to attend to their experience. (Clayton 2013, p.39)*

Reflections on the nature of Christ's presence

Thus, we return to the question with which we began in our consideration of the autonomous and buffered self (Taylor 2007). How does the practice of spiritual care in the context of limit conditions create and fashion questions for the self and the possibility of its relationship with transcendence? Does the buffered self have to be closed off from any relationship with God, or can the very dimension of tragedy and loss in the different pastoral realities described earlier themselves point to the possibility of redemption and reconciliation? Clayton himself, in writing about his contemplative stance, is inspired by a quotation from Rowan Williams: 'lives of holy wisdom are the way in which the brokenness of creation is mended' (Williams 2000, p.43).

Dan Hardy (1996, pp.86–87) has written perceptively about what it means to assert Christ's presence. In another article entitled 'The Spirit of God in creation and reconciliation' he says: 'The act of God's reconciliation is the renewal of his presence in the contextualities of existence' (Hardy 2001, p.87). God renews his being with all of creation moment by moment, and that renewal is itself an act of reconciliation. God confers on human beings what Hardy calls a 'fuller dynamic order', which is the reality of his being. This confers both a 'richer source of energy' and 'a higher quality of relationship' than the world can make available from its own resources. Together the combination of energy and relationship is that 'higher order of dynamic order' that only God can give. This abstract language is a means of speaking of the richness of divine being, but which does not simply overwhelm those who encounter God. Instead full contextuality is restored both with human beings and the natural order. Those most diminished in their lives, and therefore most decontextualised, have new life provided for them in their abandonment. This is a gift of love and God meets those who are so abandoned by providing others to care for them, and so restoring their true context. This does not remove suffering, but it holds that suffering in the presence of God. It echoes much of what Rees and Clayton were arguing earlier in this chapter. Peter Ochs, who has written a study of post-liberal Christianity and Judaism, notes that Hardy says that '*ehyey imach*', the Hebrew phrase from Exodus 3, which can be translated as 'I will be with you', belongs to God's very self-identity. Ochs argues further that this also embraces the addition of the Midrash *Exodus Rabbah* 'I will suffer with you'. Ochs reads Hardy in this way because Hardy argues that through Christ's suffering God is present with humanity in his suffering; this is also redemptive in the contingencies of our daily lives and not only at the end of time (eschatology) through the presence of the Spirit of God (pneumatology); that we are redeemed in relationship to God's unity, which is the unity of the body of Christ; that our suffering is a mark of disunity in relationship to the divine Unity; and such redemption is neither by our own works, nor by divine will working independent of our actions, but by the Spirit of God working through our actions. Such actions of God are found both in Jewish and Christian identities as they serve God in the world. While not collapsing Christianity and Judaism into one, he nevertheless sees the action of God as redemptive beyond the boundaries of church and synagogue (Hardy 2001, p.111; Ochs 2011, pp.167–195).

Chaplaincy embodies this redemptive presence of God in the face of suffering. Spiritual care, I have argued, is in fact the 'making present of Christ'. Even more, the chaplain themselves embody Christ in this making present, or in other words in their performance of spiritual care. These are large, and humbling, claims. Yet perhaps it is time that, interwoven in the necessary rhetoric of spiritual discourse and functional delivery of spiritual services as part of clinical care, the self-description of Christian chaplaincy is that it is part of the redemptive action of God's Spirit in the world. To make such claims is not to move into the old debate of the nature of priesthood or minister. It is not to make *per se* imperialist claims *vis-à-vis* other faiths, for chaplaincy must be multi-faith today. Yet it is to recall Christian chaplaincy to its true origin, that which underlies all its actions, which is the redemptive Spirit of God as it heals, reconciles and makes new in the midst of brokenness. That is the task of the chaplain, both to perform and to embody. The chaplain does so in inextricable relationship with the patient, whom she walks alongside and suffers with: *com-passio*. In so doing, such a relationship holds up an image of the spiritual self in the midst of suffering and death, and so affirms the possibility of Taylor's vision of what it means to be a person in the contemporary world.

CHAPTER 14

Assisted Suicide

A Dignified End to Severe and Enduring Mental Illness?

Charles Thody

My first full-time appointment as a mental health chaplain was in a high secure forensic psychiatric setting. I had some experience of sessional work in community mental health, but this was a completely new world to me, one of challenges and (at times) harrowing insights, yet one that gifted me invaluable insight into human nature in ways that I could not have imagined. I was privileged to be part of a team developing a completely new service, working with patients regarded as the most dangerous to society. In the years to come I was to become aware of immense acts of cruelty and, at the same time, immense acts of human kindness.

Upon taking up the appointment a colleague wrote to me, welcoming me to 'the strange yet beautiful world of mental health'. Another colleague, an experienced chaplain in a similar setting, welcomed me to the 'paradoxical world' of forensic mental health. Their words of welcome stuck in my mind throughout my work in that particular setting, and remain with me as I consider the subject of this chapter.

I came to realise that my own 'spirituality' was constantly challenged by the environment in which I worked, and (I strongly believe) was much developed and broadened by my experiences. In a sense, my own spirituality was somewhat paradoxical, and I believe it needed to be in order to understand something of the identity of the people I worked with. I entered this particular ministry with a spirituality set very much by the established church – a fairly traditional Anglican upbringing, followed by three years of training in an Anglican theological college, and a few years in quite a traditional parish ministry. As my role developed in the high secure setting, so my own beliefs and spirituality broadened immensely – I found that I changed from what might be regarded as a fairly traditional 'conservative catholic' ecclesiology, to a broad spirituality very influenced by aspects of a number of different faiths. 'Faith' became far more important, as opposed to the 'rules' of a particular faith or church tradition.

The establishment I worked in was 'home' to patients of many and varied traditions, and thus I was fortunate to have managed a department that included representatives of a number of different faiths. Between us we worked to develop a chaplaincy service that reflected the needs of such a varied community. In essence the 'normal' expected (and often traditional) boundaries of established faith communities were regularly challenged (and often fell) within the establishment we worked in, as we sought to find new ways of caring for the spiritual needs of those who were in our care. This challenge fed my own spiritual development and most certainly opened my mind to possibilities that I could not have considered had I remained a parish priest within a Church of England parish.

One such challenge was the thorny and emotional issue of assisted suicide. In both my private life and my parochial ministry, the subject had challenged me on a number of occasions. I often questioned the reasons behind seemingly keeping a person alive with medication when they clearly suffered and had no quality of life to enjoy. Why should a person suffer interminably when life could, perhaps, end in a peaceful and dignified way? Often I had heard parishioners ask these very questions, particularly those who had led very active lives to find themselves 'struck down' with a terminal illness that lasted for months, sometimes years, restricting all that made the person just who they were. I often supported people in such situations as they underwent medical treatment and yet desperately wanted to avoid such treatment and be allowed to die. As a parish priest I could only support them through the path they were experiencing, and could not condone any such feeling or wish held by the person that they simply wished to die with dignity. Support for such thoughts may have been construed as support for the notion of suicide, and surely the teachings of the churches promote sanctity of life.

On a number of occasions, I therefore found myself in tension with fellow clergy when the issue of supporting a person's desire to end their life had arisen.

My move into the world of forensic psychiatry therefore opened the possibility of exploring this issue once again, but in a very different environment and one that rarely reflected that of the parochial world from which I had come. With my own spirituality being one that needs to explore and push boundaries, one that struggles to be restricted by traditional teachings and traditions, this was an exciting opportunity. As my colleague had so eloquently described it when I took up the post, the paradoxical world of forensic mental health afforded opportunity to explore and question in ways that other forms of ministry had not really allowed.

It is with this background, of an enquiring spirituality, that I enter into the topic of this chapter. The topic of assisted suicide has been much discussed within the boundaries of general healthcare, and yet little consideration has been given within the world of mental health. For clarity, 'assisted suicide' is the action whereby a person is prescribed a lethal dose of medication by a medical professional, but administers the dose him or herself. This is quite different to the topic of euthanasia, where a person's life is ended by the direct actions of another. Within this chapter I aim to explore the possibility of assisted suicide within the world of severe and enduring mental illness. I do not aim to explore the complicated legislative issues that surround this subject, but instead (using a fictitious case study) explore issues surrounding dignity, suicide and sanctity of life. I have chosen to use this fictitious study to protect the identity of any patients that I have worked with in my work as a mental health chaplain.

My fictional patient suffers from an acute and enduring mental illness and is sectioned under the Mental Health Act (1983). She suffered considerable physical and sexual abuse from childhood and has been sentenced to life imprisonment for a violent crime. She has been resident within secure establishments for 35 years and is now in her 60s. The prospect of ever living outside of secure establishments is extremely low as her mental state fluctuates considerably and her risk to public safety remains high. She is very aware of the risk she poses to society, and does not contest this. She has made a number of attempts to end her own life, and has now requested permission to apply for assisted suicide. She regularly states that she has led an abusive and undignified life, is tormented by her past and simply wishes to be allowed to choose dignity in death.

Whilst this patient is fictional, the issues raised are very real in my experience. As a chaplain, I would first be interested in her understanding of 'dignity'. I would wish to explore whether her understanding of this may be somewhat distorted by her illness.

The Royal College of Nursing (RCN) defines dignity as being:

concerned with how people feel, think and behave in relation to the worth or value of themselves and others… Dignity applies equally to those who have capacity and to those who lack it. Everyone has equal worth as human beings and must be treated as if they are able to feel, think and behave in relation to their own worth or value. (Royal College of Nursing 2008)

This may be a much simplified definition of dignity, but is one that I believe works well when providing care for people who suffer, regardless of their illness. In all decisions made with regard to care, it is of paramount importance that the patient is recognised as having equal worth and value to the care-giver, and from this should grow a respect for the position of each within the therapeutic relationship. Yet, when it comes to the question of ending of life it appears that this view of 'dignity' is thrown into question by some ethicists.

In an article entitled 'Death with dignity', Peter Allmark questions the term 'dignity' and questions the much used phrase 'death with dignity', which he suggests is used as an emotive argument for assisted suicide. He creates an argument that suggests the concept of dignity is something that is subjective. Allmark suggests that one person's belief in what gives them dignity is different to the next, and so on, and that:

dying with dignity is whatever the dying person thinks it is. Hence, for example, if someone thinks it is undignified to die in a confused state, or incontinent, or heavily dependent on others, then it is undignified for him. (Allmark 2002, p.256)

This then presents something of a problem when considering the issue of assisted suicide. As Allmark writes,

If we were to say that assisted suicide should be an option for all people to ensure they had (subjectively) dignified deaths, we would have to provide that option to anyone who felt their current situation required it to maintain their dignity. Hence, someone who felt that impotence, or hay fever, undermined their dignity would have the same right to assisted suicide as someone who felt that way about a terminal, wasting disease. (Allmark 2002, p.256)

His argument is quite powerful. One could say that dignity is something that is pervasive, difficult to define, but is recognised in someone, something that belongs to a person as a whole rather than something specific. If this is the case, then dignity is not something that can be taken away (Allmark uses the examples of the persons of Jesus, Gandhi or Mandela, all people who suffered immensely, but never lost their dignity).

Allmark ultimately argues that the term 'death with dignity' is a weak yet emotive term, and that perhaps people really mean 'death without indignity'. Indignity, he argues, is something that is an affront on a person's naturally held dignity. Aristotelian thought would say that an essential feature of being human is the ability to reason, and that human dignity arises from this. So, it is possible that another person's actions, or a disease, threaten the ability to reason, and thus affront a person's dignity. Taking this a step further, Kantian thought would say that imposing an indignity upon a person would fail to recognise that person as an end in their own right.

So, logic therefore says that the responsibility of a healthcare professional is to recognise that every human being has dignity and thus one must not impose indignities upon a patient or, where they may be necessary (side effects of certain drugs, etc.) they should be minimised.

Ultimately Allmark argues that, as a person has an inherent dignity by the virtue of being human, then assisted suicide does nothing to improve a person's dignity and could, in fact, even be an affront to the dignity that the person holds.

So how would my mental health patient react to such views? I believe in two ways. In the first instance she would claim that indignities have been placed upon her by the 'system'. Being sectioned under the Mental Health Act (1983), feeling as if you are a 'diagnosis' rather than a person, feeling disempowered in your decision making, often lead mental health patients to feel as if they no longer have a sense of identity or being. To her, any sense of being 'human' has been stripped away, and thus any sense of personal value or worth – of 'dignity'. If this were her only response, then there would clearly be a responsibility upon those who care for her to ensure she is bestowed a sense of worth and value, personal identity and purpose. Her plea for assisted suicide would not be justified in this instance; instead the 'system' would need to examine itself and seek ways of ensuring it recognised her dignity, and bestow upon her a sense of worth and value.

Yet, it may be that the patient sees things differently. If she has been tormented mentally for many years by her condition, over which she has no control but yet is rational enough to recognise this, then she has a very strong sense of the dignity that she has lost as a result of the illness and the indignity it has imposed upon her, and indeed on other people. Her many years in secure institutions have helped her to understand her condition, and also the effect her condition has had upon others. She is desperate to end her life as she struggles to live with the torment her illness brings her, and also the pain and suffering it has brought others. Her desire to end her life is compounded by the knowledge that there is no known 'cure' for her condition and that she will, therefore, have to live the rest of her days with such torment. To her, she has lost her dignity, through the 'fault' of her illness.

Some would argue that the patient, due to her mental illness, is unable to reason and thus has no ability to make a rational argument about dignity. This is something that I would contest. From experience, I find many people who are sectioned under the Mental Health Act (1983), and suffer from enduring mental illness, are extremely capable of reason and will often have a much clearer view of a situation than others. It is also interesting to note that the Mental Capacity Act (2005) operates with the assumption that all have capacity, which is a considerable culture shift from preceding thought that effectively assumed a person with mental illness does not have capacity.

Küng puts a very good argument for the case of assisted suicide in his book, *A Dignified Dying* (1995). In his essay he reflects upon the situation of his brother who died very painfully from a long-term incurable illness. Küng approaches his argument from a Christian perspective and asks (of the suffering he witnessed in his brother), 'Is this the death that God gives, that God ordains?' (Küng 1995, p.25).

As a chaplain from a Christian tradition, this is a question I must consider. In the case of Küng's brother, a painful death was inevitable, and it was known that death would soon come. So, it does seem right to me that Küng and his family wished assisted suicide for him, to relieve him of his awful suffering. Yet could I ask the same question in the case of my mental health patient? The difficulty in this instance is the condition the patient is in. She suffers terrible mental torment, yet this torment alone is not going to bring about her death. Or is it? Controversially, one could say it is highly likely that it will, as it brings such a strong desire within her to commit suicide, a desire that, arguably, would not be there without the illness. As there is no known medication to treat her condition, it could also be argued that her torment is simply going to become worse as time goes on.

Küng's view is that humans are given freedom by God in life, and so that also means we are given freedom in decision making about the end of our lives. Whilst he goes to great pains to point out that any such decisions should be made with the utmost responsibility, conscience, social understanding and the effect the decision would have upon others, he says, 'No one should be forced into going on living at all costs' (Küng 1995, p.31). And

> *If God makes the whole of life a human responsibility, then this responsibility also applies to the last phase of our lives, indeed it applies even more to the real emergency of our lives, when it is a matter of dying. Why should this last phase of life in particular be exempted from responsibility? (Küng 1995, p.38)*

Whilst Küng is writing from the experience of witnessing a death from terminal illness, his ethic must surely remain regardless of the illness that is experienced. Of course, the argument that would be placed against this is the 'sanctity of life' argument.

There are, of course, views opposed to those of Küng and others, and I suggest that many opposed views arise from the churches' discussions around the emotive issue of suicide. As part of his discussion about this, and the relationship between suicide and assisted suicide, Crawford asks, 'What is the use of prolonging an existence which is full of pain and distress when death could release? On a utilitarian basis, the death would bring relief to the sufferer and benefit to the relatives' (Crawford 1991, p.30).

Until 1961 suicide was still a criminal offence in the UK, and the force behind such views was the churches. Taking one's own life was (and still is, according to many Christians) regarded as an offence against the divine right of God, and thus a sin. With the repeal of that law in 1961, Crawford suggests that to rule assisted suicide as illegal is simply illogical, as ultimately it is the sufferer who chooses to take away their life and is responsible for the action of doing so.

Within his discussion, Crawford (1991) asks the reader to imagine they are an older person who is told that at 80 years old they will have the opportunity to die a peaceful death, yet if they choose to stay alive beyond their 80th birthday they will die a painful and suffering death some days later. He asks the reader, 'what would you do?' (1991, p.49). He suggests that by far the majority would choose to die a peaceful death at 80 and quotes Matthew 7:12 'So whatever you wish that men would do to you, do so to them; for this is the law and the prophets'.

Crawford's argument continues: 'Life is not to be preserved at all costs, for death is not to be feared. It is a transition, not a terminus. Compassion and love can override commandments, as shown by the ministry of Jesus' (1991, p.49).

If, as a Christian, I do not fear death then why should I be concerned about the 'premature' ending of life if such an ending relieves intolerable suffering? Of course, not all agree with this stance. Bloch and Heyd discuss the ethic of suicide in *Psychiatric Ethics* (2009). They quote Kant, who very clearly supports an absolute prohibition to suicide on the grounds of rational argument. According to Kant, we have a duty to ourselves to choose life over death, and he presents the maxim,

> *'From self-love I make it my principle to shorten my life if its continuance threatens more evil than it promises pleasure' could never become a 'universal law of nature'. This is due to the fact that the function of self-love is 'the furtherance of life' and it would contradict itself if it led to annihilation. (Bloch and Heyd 2009, p.233)*

I suggest that this argument expresses fear of suicide simply becoming a normally accepted aspect of life, and the beginnings of the so called 'slippery slope' argument against assisted suicide. Bloch and Heyd then apply this thinking to a clinical situation, where a 26-year-old woman, incapacitated by cerebral palsy and a voluntary patient on a psychiatric ward in North America, refused food and sought a court order to stop staff force feeding her. The court ruled in favour of the hospital, taking the view that her 'assisted suicide' (assisted because the hospital would have stopped feeding her) would have a devastating effect upon the other patients in the institution. So, not only does a Kantian ethic appear to rule against any form of assisted suicide, a Utilitarian one does also, as this court ruling takes into account what it sees as the common or greater good. Indeed, Bloch and Heyd conclude by writing, 'Even if a person should have the freedom to commit suicide…it does not follow that the civic community has the responsibility to assist anyone in that act of suicide' (2009, p.242).

So, in this argument, the primacy of the common good must override the private interest. This is a very Utilitarian approach, and one with considerable weight, but one with which I remain considerably uncomfortable.

Badham presents a balanced argument in favour of euthanasia from a Christian point of view. In his case, he suggests that changing attitudes within the churches with regard to medical intervention over the years point to the fact that the churches' ethical attitudes do change. Years ago, churches taught that the use of medicine was tantamount to sorcery and any form of surgery was forbidden. In 1829, Pope Leo XII declared that anyone who chose to be vaccinated against smallpox was 'no longer a child of God' (Badham 1996, p.103) as smallpox was a judgement of God and thus vaccination was a challenge to heaven!

Badham suggests that the arguments used against assisted suicide by the churches are the same arguments that were used in history against the development of medicine and so there is a sense that the churches choose an argument to meet their needs at the time.

With regard to the taking of one's own life, I am more at ease with Badham's approach. He believes it is a myth that the Bible says one is not to take one's own life. Indeed he cites a number of examples where the taking of one's own life is condoned in the Judaic/Christian scriptures – mentioning Samson, King Saul and his armour bearer and Judas. Badham then comments upon what a number of writers have named 'Jesus' Golden Rule' quoted from John 15:13, 'Greater love has no man than this, than to lay down his life for his friends.' He also quotes Ecclesiasticus 30:17, which reads 'Death is better than a miserable life, end eternal rest than chronic sickness' (Badham 1996, p.107).

So it would seem that the sanctity of life argument is not watertight and is, perhaps, a more traditional argument against difficult subjects like assisted suicide. Returning to Crawford, in concluding his discussion about suicide and assisted suicide, he writes, 'Suicide does not involve another person, wither friend or doctor, but euthanasia does and therefore is more complex' (1991, p.51). This comment highlights the continued difficulty with this whole issue. With assisted suicide, the person wishing to die takes the action to end their life, others are involved and thus, it could be argued, do have some responsibility as they are providing the means. However, I believe one has to think more widely than this. From personal experience as a chaplain, I have experienced the devastation a patient's suicide causes their peers and the medical staff who have cared for them. If a patient, such as my fictitious patient from earlier, is so tormented by their condition that they will go to any lengths to take their own life, then their distress at making several 'failed' attempts is hard to bear, for both them and the staff.

If I return, therefore, to the discussion about dignity, it could be strongly argued that, for someone like my patient who has the act of suicide at the forefront of her mind every day, assisted suicide (after very careful consideration) would afford her dignity. She would have the opportunity to prepare herself for a peaceful and non-violent death, after properly informed decision and perhaps with people alongside her who care for her. Thus, her sense of value and worth would be intact.

Naudts *et al.* (2006) point out that, in 2002, Belgium became unique in allowing assisted suicide for those who suffer from mental illness. The words of the act state that, 'The patient should be in a medically hopeless condition of constant and unbearable physical or mental suffering, which cannot be cured and which is a consequence of a severe and incurable disorder caused by accident or disease' (Naudts *et al.* 2006, p.405).

Within psychiatry the treatability of certain mental disorders is debated. In particular, diagnosis of personality disorders is controversial, and they have historically been widely regarded as untreatable. Would this then make a patient with a severe personality disorder acceptable for assisted suicide should they apply for it? Many would say, 'No', as there is much still to learn about the disorder and it may yet prove to be treatable. However, my question is, 'How does this relate to permissions given for assisted suicide for a patient who has terminal cancer?' It may be that, in the present, there is no cure for terminal cancer, but the future is unpredictable and a cure could be discovered at any time. Yet support has grown for the legalisation of assisted suicide for patients with terminal illness, so why not with a mental illness that, as yet, has no known cure?

I believe there to be a *fundamental* inequality if the ethic of assisted suicide is more acceptable for those with physical suffering than mental suffering. If one were to approach this from a narrative ethics point of view, one would listen to the story of the patient and look beyond the diagnosis to the value of the patient's story. As Martinez (2009) writes, 'In a narrative approach, diagnosis is secondary to acknowledging the patient as someone with a story to tell, who requires support for their voice to be effectively heard' (Martinez 2009, p.56).

In the case of my patient, she would have a very powerful story to tell of her suffering and torment, and would feel that she is not listened to. Why would this be? Primarily because the role of the psychiatric healthcare system is to 'advocate for the vulnerable, disabled and infirm of society and, when necessary, to protect them from themselves or others. A classic prevention of this task is prevention of suicide' (Naudts *et al.* 2006, p.407).

If she felt listened to, and her genuinely held plea for assisted suicide was accepted (rather than immediately being told it is simply not allowed), she would have a sense of value and worth, and thus dignity, that she has not experienced for some time. Indeed, she may not even progress to the act of assisted suicide and may well live more comfortably with her torment, in the knowledge that those who care for her do share her concern and understand her point of view.

In a memo to the House of Lords in August 2004, the Swiss organisation Dignitas points out that less than 20 per cent of its members who have received the 'green light' (that is have been accepted after due consideration for assisted suicide) actually go ahead with the act. The great majority report that being delivered 'from their dilemma either to be forced to follow the path through hell of their suffering or to intend a high risk suicide attempt on their own' (Dignitas 2004, para 30) brings psychological relief and strengthens them to carry on, knowing they do have an option available to them.

In conclusion, I acknowledge that the ethical issue of assisted suicide is complex and incredibly emotive. Yet I still seek to support the ethic that is so often shied away from, that assisted suicide could bring a dignified end to severe and enduring mental illness and should not be ruled out. I have not sought to discuss the legislation required, or the safeguards that would, undoubtedly and rightly, need to be in place to allow for assisted suicide in a mental health setting. These issues alone warrant considerably more study than afforded in this chapter. But I do believe that the ethic itself does warrant further attention, and its acceptance would be beneficial to many who feel they must end their own lives because of their mental torment. I am concerned that much energy is spent on discussing the issues of legislation, to the detriment of discussion of the ethic itself.

I began this chapter reflecting upon a paradoxical spirituality that leads me to explore such issues. I recall, many years ago (whilst training in theological college) attending a baptism on Easter Saturday. As joyful as the occasion was, I could not fail to be drawn by a very powerful rood screen with a simple but graphic depiction of the crucifixion carved above it. This particular depiction seemed (to me at least) to tell the story 'as it was', with no attempts to sanitise or glorify. It depicted what I saw then (and continue to see) as the paradox of that scene – awful suffering combined with love and compassion: the suffering of the Christ figure on the cross, yet the love that somehow radiated through that suffering, the sanctity of life and the sanctity of death.

Alongside was depicted the suffering and yet love and compassion of those close to him, his mother and the disciple, who must have longed for him to live, yet also understood the death and stood by him when others ran away.

It seems to me that a spirituality that seeks to be open to the sanctity and suffering of life and death cannot fail to hold compassion at its heart. If this is so, then such spirituality will be open to possibilities such as assisted suicide (and such other possibilities that may be generally regarded as 'taboo' by traditional teaching). Life is not perfect and suffering is a harsh reality for many (both physical and mental) – should this suffering be endured? Does God desire such suffering? I, for one, cannot believe that he does. I maintain that, in this imperfect life, there are times when it is right to yield to possibilities such as assisted suicide, and in doing so, trust in the love and mercy of God. The image and event of the crucifixion so powerfully illustrate this to me, to my fictitious patient and to so many like her whom I have met in real life.

CHAPTER 15

Insights into Spiritual Need and Care Arising Out of the Experience of Those Living with Mild Cognitive Impairment (MCI)

Richard Wharton

Introduction to Mild Cognitive Impairment and research project

In this chapter I examine what can be learnt from the experiences of those living with Mild Cognitive Impairment (MCI) about our understandings of personhood and some of the implications of these understandings for those offering spiritual care. These reflections emerged from a piece of qualitative research carried out as part of a Master's degree programme through St Michael's College, Llandaff in 2012, under the supervision of an experienced healthcare chaplain. The research participants were all receiving care from a Midlands-based mental health NHS Trust. At the time of writing, I work as a chaplain in the Queen Elizabeth Hospital Birmingham (QEHB), part of University Hospitals Birmingham NHS Foundation Trust (UHBFT).

Empirical research (e.g. Albert *et al.* 2011; Ritchie, Arturo and Touchon 2001) has shown that a significant number of people who live with MCI go on to develop dementia. The yearly rates of conversion from MCI to different forms of dementia vary from 10–15 per cent (Alzheimer's Society 2008) to as much as 53 per cent (Ritchie *et al.* 2001) in people aged 60 or over. In part, these discrepancies may be due to the fact that 'there is still no common consensus on diagnostic criteria' (Ritchie *et al.* 2001, p.37). As Ritchie *et al.* point out, the absence of neurological tests is 'a major shortcoming of current MCI criteria' (2001, p.40). Studies show that MCI is commonly associated with significant morbidity, economic hardship and distress to care-givers (Garand *et al.* 2005), as well as emotional, cognitive and behavioural decline (Feldman *et al.* 2004).

The impact that MCI has upon an individual's sense of self emphasises the need for a multi-disciplinary and multi-dimensional approach to care (Kitwood 1997; McSherry 2006; Shamy 2003; Swinton 2001, 2008; White 2006). Effective holistic care of those with mental illness necessitates as much an understanding of their social narrative, spirituality, values and connectedness, as it does of their neuropathology.

One particular focus within the holistic care literature is the relationship between personhood and mental health. Swinton (2008), for example, draws attention to the prevailing liberal worldview which suggests that those living with dementia are somehow incomplete people. He remarks that such a view 'venerates a specific set of capacities, values, assumptions and expectations: the primacy of reason, rationality, cognitive ability, independence and the capacity for self-advocacy' (2008, p.22). He continues, saying that 'personhood is defined precisely by those aspects of experience that people with dementia lose as their condition progresses' (2008, p.22), and is highly critical of the view that personhood is defined by such functionality, by which the sufferer is inevitably depersonalised. Swinton draws attention to the way in which Tom Kitwood shifts our understanding of personhood away from such functionality. Kitwood writes that personhood, 'is a standing or status that is bestowed upon one human being, by others, in the context of relationship and social being' (1997, p.8). In other words, to be a person is to exist in relationship. Swinton asserts that personhood is 'a gift of community' (2008, p.27).

Given the connections between holistic care, mental health, personhood and spirituality, it is reasonable to suggest that those who have been diagnosed with MCI (and who live with the prospect of decreasing mental capacity and the possibility of developing dementia), may have identifiable and distinctive spiritual needs that could be helpfully understood.

Exploring spirituality in healthcare

Whilst much has been written from both spiritual and nursing care perspectives about the spiritual needs of people with dementia in its various forms and stages, no specific research appears to have been conducted that enquires about the spiritual needs of those living with MCI. What impact, for instance, might the prospect of decreasing mental capacity and increased memory impairment have upon an individual's perceived sense that they are a whole person, autonomous, yet integrated in social, religious or historical contexts? How might changes in self-image, or how might the prospect of impaired capacity affect their self-esteem and readiness to engage within these and other networks?

With the hope of being able to clarify the distinctive contribution that spirituality and spiritual care can offer to the multi-disciplinary team, I set out to explore, from a spiritual care perspective, the lived experience of Christian patients who had been diagnosed with MCI. I paid attention particularly to the impact that memory impairment had upon their sense of self – their personhood and their spiritual well being.

My original study therefore sought to develop theories about whether people from a Christian background living with MCI had distinctive, identifiable spiritual needs.

Defining spirituality for healthcare

Identifying the spiritual needs of any particular group of patients will necessitate a robust definition of what spirituality is in the first place. Therefore, and mindful that spirituality cannot solely be defined from the perspective of organised religion, I adopted the following humanist-phenomenological (non-religious) definition of spirituality proposed by Elkins *et al.* in 1988 as a basis for this research:

> *Spirituality…is a way of being and experiencing that comes about through awareness of a transcendent dimension and that is characterised by certain identifiable values in regard to self, others, nature, life and whatever one considers to be the Ultimate. (Elkins et al. 1988, p.10)*

Whilst not seeking to invalidate religion or to be antireligious in any sense, Elkins *et al.* explain that they 'have striven for an enlarged definition of spirituality that would not equate it with narrow religious beliefs, rituals and practices' (1988, p.8). They speak of their research participants having an awareness or understanding of nine major components:

1. a transcendent dimension
2. meaning and purpose in life
3. mission in life
4. the sacredness of life
5. material values
6. altruism
7. idealism
8. an awareness of the tragic
9. the fruits of spirituality.

If, as Elkins *et al.* suggest, spirituality is concerned with 'being and experiencing', it follows that spiritual need may become most evident when an individual's sense of who they are, their personhood, is compromised or threatened.

Research methodology

From the outset, I sought to choose the most appropriate methodological approach for this research project. The research question called for an exploration of the lived experiences of those diagnosed with MCI from a spiritual care perspective. I wanted to pay particular attention to data that demonstrated the research participants' interpretations of, and responses to their lived experiences.

This research was carried out with the support of the Birmingham Memory Assessment and Advisory Service (BMAAS), which is responsible for diagnosing and signposting individuals with MCIs in Birmingham. Those BMAAS clients who responded to the invitation to participate in this study were interviewed in their homes and consented to those interviews being recorded and transcribed anonymously.

Swinton and Mowat (2006) comment that qualitative research 'assumes that humans are by definition "interpretive creatures"; that the ways in which we make sense of the world and our experiences within it involves a constant process of interpretation and meaning-making' (2006, p.29). Licqurish and Seibold (2011) argue that qualitative research makes the assumption that meaning is constructed through engagement with the world, and therefore the 'truth' that emerges from that engagement is relative, and the meaning flexible (Licqurish and Seibold 2011, p.12).

In discerning which research methodology I was to use, it seemed particularly significant that I wanted both to explore hitherto unexplored territory (regarding MCI and spiritual need), and to ensure that any theories that emerged were rigorous and as true to the research participants' interpretive experience as possible. Grounded Theory (GT) proved itself to be the best fit for this particular enquiry.

With these factors in mind, a constructivist approach to my interpretation of the data that emerged was implied. Kathy Charmaz commented that 'constructivists study how – and sometimes why – participants construct meanings and actions in specified situations' (2006, p.130). Thus, my intention was to develop an interpretation of the data that emerged from the participants' own understanding of their lives, as opposed to one that was based upon objective explanation. Fundamental to Charmaz's understanding of constructivist GT is an understanding that the researcher's interpretation is central to the research process. As the researcher, I saw myself as an essential element in the interpretive process. It became clear that I could not 'bracket' out my own influence and bias from that process as would be the norm in positivist methodologies (Laverty 2003).

Charmaz assumes 'that neither data nor theories are discovered. Rather, we are part of the world we study and the data we collect. We construct our grounded theories through our past and present involvements and interactions with people, perspectives and research practices' (2006, p.10). Consequently, it was as if I acted as a co-creator (Swinton and Mowat 2006, p.61) of the theories that emerged.

Critical reflection

In this study I recognised a distinction between spiritual *need, inclination* and *capacity*. Whilst suggesting that a particular spiritual *need* may become most evident when, for example, an individual's sense of who they are is challenged, by spiritual *inclination* and spiritual *capacity*, I was referring respectively to, either a recognisable *pattern of behaviour*, or a recognisable *aptitude* that wasn't necessarily a spiritual *need* as such, but something that may be suggestive of one.

Three key themes, or 'theoretical categories' (Charmaz 2006, p.63), were identified throughout this research; namely, *the importance of community, the importance of control and order* and *the importance of mission and purpose.* It soon became apparent that the nine key components of spirituality, referred to by Elkins *et al.* (1988) may be limited, particularly in relation to matching the first two of these themes.

In this section I will describe selected details of these themes, holding them alongside literature from the fields of *spiritual care in a healthcare context* and of the *Christian spiritual life.* I will reflect upon some of the questions these themes raise for those offering spiritual, religious and pastoral care (particularly in an acute healthcare setting) to people living with MCI, and that may also be applicable in other contexts.

The importance of community

The experiences of all of the participants in this research demonstrated the importance of community in both shaping and affirming their identity and well-being. They did this in three distinct ways, two of which I will reflect on here: in demonstrating evidence of *the importance of their origins and inspirations,* and of *the importance of their sense of belonging.*

One research participant, 'Averyl', described how, as the second of three children, she was dependent upon the charity of religious sisters for her education. She described how this early experience affected her perception of wealth and poverty, and the relationship between rich and poor. She said, 'My family benefitted from that attitude of the Sisters, I knew what it was about, I knew that it wasn't theoretic for me... I had seen it, I had experience, I gained from it.'

Throughout Averyl's interview, she returned repeatedly in her responses to this critically formative period of her young life. She did this in ways that suggested these experiences not only shaped her younger life, but that they continued to inform her sense of who she was.

Janet Ruffing (2011), writing about the practice of spiritual direction in the Christian tradition, comments that 'creating an internal narrative is the way we maintain a sense of continuity of ourselves through time' (2011, p.68). Speaking of 'transformative experiences' that fundamentally alter an individual's vision of reality (such as this expressed by Averyl), Ruffing argues that narratives are required 'that can integrate past and future' (2011, p.72). Stephen Crites (1971), reflecting upon this narrative quality of experience, argues that such stories are in fact 'sacred' in so far as people's 'sense of self and world is created through them…they live, so to speak, in the arms and legs and bellies of the celebrants' (1971, p.295). So much so, he argues, that they may carry the authority of scripture for those whose lives are immersed there, '[creating] a world of consciousness and the self that is oriented to it' (1971, p.296).

As a healthcare chaplain currently working in a large acute teaching hospital, this raises a number of pertinent questions:

1. How could these 'transformative', sacred narratives of our patients be given opportunity to play a more creative role – through story-telling and reminiscence work (e.g. MacKinlay 2006, p.81ff) in shaping people's experience of healing, and in restoring a sense of well-being?

2. How might this understanding of 'transformative experience' enrich the healthcare practitioner's assessment of, and response to, the spiritual needs of their patients? What opportunities might this create for working creatively across the multi-disciplinary team as they engage in psycho-social and spiritual care?

3. In a culture where individualism and rights to privacy are heralded as virtues, what might an awareness of the potency of story-sharing have upon how we design the arrangements of our inpatient wards?

All of the participants in this study were eager to sustain and strengthen existing social networks to which they could meaningfully contribute. In his *Becoming Human* (1999) Jean Vanier wrote:

> *What is this need to belong? Is it only a way of dealing with personal insecurity, sharing in the sense of identity that a group provides? Or is this sense of belonging an important part of everyone's journey to freedom?… My vision is that belonging should be at the heart of a fundamental discovery: that we all belong to a common humanity, the human race. (1999, p.36)*

Vanier continues, 'we do not discover who we are, we do not reach true humanness, in a solitary state, we discover it through mutual dependency, in weakness, in learning through belonging' (1999, p.41). This resonates with the inherently compassionate African virtue of Ubuntu. Archbishop Desmond Tutu writes, '[Ubuntu] means my humanity is caught up, inextricably bound up, in theirs... We say, "a person is a person through other people"... I am human because I belong' (1999, pp.34–35).

One research participant, Averyl, explained that whilst she maintained her independence in a variety of ways, she was *dependent* upon other members of the religious community to which she belonged for an affirmation of her self-image. Similarly, 'Connie' spoke of the increase in self-confidence she experienced (after her diagnosis of MCI) due to a heightening sense of shared responsibility in relation to a social community group, which worked to tackle the problem of isolation amongst elders in her local community. 'Dee' experienced a similar reciprocity through community engagement. Her sense of belonging in a dance group grew when she found the courage to attend classes in which she was both taught, and eventually also taught others.

These experiences raise three further questions:

1. In the offering of pastoral/spiritual care, how much attention is given to where our patients derive a sense of belonging, and how might this information, appropriately shared, enrich attempts (through, for example, focused activity programmes in ward environments) to create opportunities for healing and wholeness?

2. What creative links and partnerships could be developed between healthcare providers and community organisations and groups to enhance healing and wholeness (cf. Kennedy *et al.* 2013)?

3. How might these links be developed to ensure the safer discharge of vulnerable patients from hospital (particularly when they are not able to return to their previous home), and in order that any possible disruption to an individual's sense of belonging is minimised?

Vanier suggests that 'belonging is the fulcrum point for the individual between a sense of self and a sense of society' (1999, p.57). In other words, it is through belonging that an individual may begin to gain greater self-awareness, or discover their 'real self', and likewise it is through the discovery of their 'real self' that they can better understand their place in community.

The importance of control and order

Another significant characteristic of all those interviewed for this research was how they developed strategies to enhance a sense of control and order in response to their memory impairments. These strategies appeared to be employed to help them to *sustain or protect* a sense of self – their personhood (see also Gauthier *et al.* 2006, p.1267; Lu, Haase and Farran 2007, p.82).

Whilst reflecting upon how these strategies might be understood, I was drawn to a concept (adopted from earlier psychological research) developed by Anne Deveson in her work, *Resilience* (2003) (see also Lloyd 2006, 2011). In the light of living through the trauma of both the suicide of her son and death of her partner, Deveson describes *resilience* as 'a life force' that prompts 'regeneration and renewal' (2003, p.267), and 'the ability to confront adversity and still find hope and meaning in life' (2003, p.2). Benson and Thistlethwaite suggest that 'resilience may be conceptualised as reflecting the positive capacity of a person to bounce back from adverse events such as conflict or failure, and to learn from positive events such as increased responsibility' (2008, p.88). Through the use of a variety of strategies, all of the participants in this study appeared to be increasing their resilience to the impact of their memory impairments.

One resilience-building strategy, employed by all of the participants in this study, was extensive participation in religious rituals (e.g. formal acts of prayer, reading of scriptures, sacraments and worship) and social rituals (e.g. rituals of family routines and shared community activities). Benson and Thistlethwaite (2008) acknowledge that the practice of using ritual is amongst the numerous factors affecting resilience and mental health (2008, p.89). One way of understanding such use of (particularly religious) ritual was offered by Viktor Frankl (1984) who suggested that 'being human always points, and is directed, to something, or someone, other than oneself' (1984, p.115). He refers to the concept of 'the self-transcendence of human existence' (1984, p.115) to describe this aspect of human nature. Elizabeth MacKinlay (2006) suggests that human beings need the symbolism that ritual provides 'to connect us with meanings too deep to be expressed in words' (2006, p.132).

These points raise further questions for those responding to the spiritual needs of those living with MCI in healthcare settings:

1. How can a sense of control and order be sustained for those living with MCI or other mental health-related conditions in an inpatient healthcare setting where so much choice, power, freedom of movement and independence is lost?

2. Whilst an awareness of 'self-transcendence', or a sense of connection with God may be encouraged, for example, through religious ritual and formal prayer, in what ways might non-religious rituals be used in a healthcare setting to enhance resilience?

One of the complex challenges to maintaining a sense of self through seeking control and order in life that was significant for all of the participants in this study was that there was a variety of ways in which they grappled with *dichotomy*. By dichotomy, I am referring to particular personality traits or experiences that seem to contradict each other, but that continued to be held in tensive relationship with each other.

Over the past few decades within the Christian spiritual tradition, there has been a resurgence of interest in exploring the notion that there are recognisable stages of faith development (e.g. Fowler 1981; Rohr 2011). Fowler refers to the fifth of his seven stages of faith development as *Conjunctive Faith* (1981, pp.184ff). He describes this as:

> *a way of seeing, of knowing, of committing [that] moves beyond the dichotomising logic of stage 4's 'either/or.' It sees both (or many) sides of an issue simultaneously... Conjunctive faith involves going beyond the explicit ideological system and clear boundaries of identity that Stage 4 worked so hard to construct and to adhere to. (1981, pp.185–186)*

Whilst caution needs to be exercised in drawing a parallel between the conscious relinquishing of power implied by Fowler and the involuntary loss of power experienced by those I interviewed living with MCI, it was interesting to recognise a similar acknowledgement of living with dichotomous experiences and uncertain boundaries. Examples revealed in the study included the participants' dual senses of '*dependence – independence*', '*confidence – feelings of insecurity*', '*true self – persona self*', '*success – failure*' and '*power – weakness*'.

This grappling with dichotomy does not appear to me to be so much a search for the 'meaning and purpose in life' that Elkins *et al.* referred to in their research (1988). Instead it seems to indicate a more fundamental search for an identity of self. It asks 'who *am* I?', rather than 'what am I to *do*?', or 'what is the *meaning* of my life?' The primary concern seems to be around '*being*', rather than '*doing*'. This question, and the discussion about living with dichotomy, seems to cast a particular light upon the apparent importance of control and order. If, as the Christian spiritual tradition acknowledges, powerlessness, ambiguity and even weakness are positively part and parcel of spiritual development and maturity, the idea of 'maintaining a sense of control and order' seems out of place. In terms of spiritual *need*, what is suggested by the tradition here is that it is possible for a new relationship to be found with this perceived need (i.e. 'control and order'), even to the extent that for some, in a positive sense, the 'need' may be relinquished.

The importance of mission and purpose

The vulnerabilities that arose from each of the participants' memory impairments appeared to be a source of inspiration for them in shaping a purposeful and meaningful engagement in their local community settings. Examples of such engagement include the decisions by one participant to remain living in an environment where she could continue to 'be of use', rather than moving to a family home, as well as a commitment to sharing in the life of prayer of her local religious community. Another participant demonstrated a strong sense of duty to local elders through her taking initiatives and responsibilities in the running of a local social community group. A third participant spoke of his sense of 'injustice' about how older people are sometimes treated, and how this sense appeared to have been heightened by his own vulnerability brought about through his memory impairments. Further, it influenced him in making specific efforts, not made previously, to listen to and include those individuals in decisions relating to the running of a community health association. How might this new engagement be understood, and what does it offer to the participants in this study?

One theme I noticed in the experiences described is that these examples of self-motivated and purposeful engagement ('mission') in such activities appear to have emerged from a pre-existent *sense of belonging*. Vanier (1999) remarks that 'society is the place where we learn our potential and become competent... It is the place where each can accomplish his or her mission' (1999, p.57). Further, he remarks that society is the place 'we need in order to live and to act in society in justice...and to take initiatives in working with others' (1999, p.59). It may be that for these participants, such purposeful engagement generates a welcomed reminder of 'competence', or of 'being taken seriously by others' in the face of their increased memory impairment.

In his reflection upon the psychological needs of those living with dementia, Kitwood (1997) identifies practical, community engagement as a significant motivating force in itself. He writes, 'to be occupied means to be involved in the process of life in a way that is personally significant, and which draws on a person's abilities and powers... If people are deprived of occupation their abilities begin to atrophy and self-esteem drains away' (1997, p.83). Seen in this way, such purposeful engagement could be viewed as much as a deliberate *strategy* to ensure that self-esteem is maintained or to mitigate against the effects of memory impairment specifically, as much as it could be seen as a result of a particular inspiration or vocation.

A second theme that emerges from these examples is that of *generosity*. Averyl's commitment to the 'service of other people', 'Betty's' support (financial and emotional) for vulnerable members of her family, and the time, skill and energy that Connie invested in a local community group for elders each demonstrate a high degree of generosity.

During the time I was reflecting upon this trend within the data, I read a report on a piece of research into the lived experience of spirituality and dementia. Padmaprabha Dalby (2011) identified in the experience of patients living with dementia, a 'common emphasis upon generosity and helping others as part of their spiritual life' (Dalby 2011, p.64). Bearing in mind the conversion rates between MCI and dementia (see earlier), I found the thematic similarity between *mission and purpose* identified in this study, and the *generosity* theme in Dalby's work intriguing. Dalby notes that other studies into the experience of those living with dementia also affirm 'that helping others or being of use to others was a key strategy in helping people to retain continuity in their lives and support their sense of self' (2011, p.72).

These observations give rise to a critical question pertinent to those working in acute healthcare settings. If mission, purposeful engagement and generosity are fundamental features of what it means to be a person, how can those working in acute care settings create opportunities for such engagement to be lived out?

Conclusion

In setting out to examine whether any connections could be made between the lived experiences of living with MCI, how we understand personhood and how those understandings affect the shape of spiritual care, some clear themes have emerged. In my reflection upon the importance of *community* it became clear that all of the research participants experienced how, perhaps unsurprisingly, a heightened sense of the importance of their origins, belonging and early transformative experiences shaped their sense of self. My understanding of this sense of self was deepened through an appreciation of the potency of resilience-building strategies, as well as through a surprisingly enhanced capacity to grapple with dichotomy in my exploration of the importance of *control and order*. Finally, in my reflection upon the importance of *mission and purpose*, I uncovered a strong inclination in the experiences of those living with MCI to engage deeply and generously in community activities.

CHAPTER 16

'A Hidden Wholeness'

Spiritual Care in a Children's Hospice

Mark Clayton

Introduction

This chapter explores chaplaincy and spiritual care in children's hospice and paediatric palliative care by investigating the connected themes of wholeness, holiness and healing, which derive in their etymology from the same root word. Writing in *The Lancet*, Liben, Papadatou and Wolfe (2008) observe that 'the task in paediatric palliative care is to help the child and their loved ones find their way as far as they can along this continuum from suffering to wholeness'; this may not be the only goal, though, but 'a frame of reference as to what may be possible, even if only partially realised' (p.858). From a clinical viewpoint, wholeness is a central objective, even in the absence of a cure. It is also central to spiritual care, and the idea of 'a hidden wholeness' comes from some words by Thomas Merton who observes that it is present 'in all visible things' as a 'mysterious unity and integrity' (McDonnell 1989, p.506). Wholeness, then, is a unifying focus of care, and, as we will see, is often represented by the shape of a circle. At the same time, spiritual care must always be mindful that serious illness in children raises questions about the attainment of wholeness. This is borne out by Mattie Stepanek, an American poet and Roman Catholic, who died just before his 14th birthday from a rare form of muscular dystrophy, and whose questions reveal the challenge of keeping such wholeness in view:

> *My life / Is not how / I planned it to be*
> *Is not how / I want it to be;*
> *Is not how / I pray for it / To be...*

Is it possible for me / To climb to such heights?
To rebuild the bridges? / To find my salvation?
(Macauley and Hylton Rushton 2012, p.130)

For many who knew him, though, Mattie's life and poetry revealed an authenticity and integration that were remarkable for his age; and, taken with his courageous questioning and vulnerability, these qualities help us to approach the concept of holiness, which we understand here in terms of the many, varied and surprising faces of love. For chaplaincy and spiritual care, practised in the Christian tradition, Mattie's vulnerability and questioning take us to the heart of a role that draws its inspiration from the humility and holiness of Jesus, who emptied himself, making himself nothing, and became obedient even to death (Phil 2:5–8). A circle is a compelling image of this, for, as Johnston (1995) observes, 'the circle is a symbol of God and a symbol of nothing' (p.170): it contains mere emptiness, and yet this is encompassed by a circumference without beginning or end. This work is rooted in contemplative disciplines such as meditation, which Freeman (1999) has described as 'practising dying', since we 'die' to the emptiness of the false, egoistic self, so that a true and more fully whole, or holy, self can slowly unfurl. In the hospice, chaplaincy seeks to acknowledge what Puchalski (2006) calls 'the inherent mystery of life' (p.x); it aims at an integration of dying and living, so that, just as Jesus washed the feet of his disciples, it is not just about end-of-life care, but includes ordinary, everyday forms of service: not the least of these are being gentle or vulnerable with others, and available to laugh, as well as sometimes cry, with them.

Our role as chaplains is often to participate in the healing dimension of palliative care, as an example from my own experience illustrates. A little Sikh baby called Pooran, who was a twin, was referred to us, having been diagnosed antenatally with a rare condition that signified a very short life expectancy. He lived for two days, before a colleague and I brought him to the hospice, where he was able to stay in a specially cooled bedroom until his funeral. Pulled between caring for their newborn daughter and their thoughts for her brother, his parents came to spend several hours with him, which enabled them to stay with the reality of his death. What also appeared to help the healing process was Pooran's footprints being painted on a circular plate, together with those of his sister Daiya, and their names written alongside the prints. A colleague of mine, who is an artist, worked with the family to make this very moving image. In its own way, it represented the 'hidden wholeness' of the babies' relationship and identity as twins both before birth and for two days afterwards. My part in this was to work with our team in welcoming and accompanying the family on this stage of their journey, before going with them to the funeral; and by doing this, it was also about affirming the hospice's healing work at the threshold of life and death.

Part one: Wholeness in the context of holistic care

Chaplaincy and spiritual care have a valid and creative place in this context, because paediatric palliative care aspires to be holistic. The World Health Organization (WHO 2014) defines such care as 'the active total care of the child's body, mind and spirit, and also involves giving support to the family'; and what is notable here is not just the reference to the 'spirit', but also the word, 'total'. The aspiration is to care for the whole person in a way that is all-encompassing, from the time of diagnosis, through the illness and into bereavement. It is represented visually on the cover of the *Oxford Textbook of Palliative Care for Children* (2012), in the form of a circular ring of small stone pebbles. The circle conveys a sense of the child and family being enfolded in a protective embrace, which will hold and keep them safe, whatever happens. A further example of the importance of this, cited by Liben *et al.* (2008), is the statement by 17-year-old Rachel, who said she wanted to die 'surrounded by friends and family, and surrounded by people that knew how to take care of her' (p.858). Chaplains need to appreciate the significance of care that is holistic. When I asked Emma, a mum who was making her first stay at the hospice, how it was going, she said that, after seven weeks in hospital with Ava, her baby daughter, it was just nice to be together with her two young sons and husband again; after that long separation, it meant a lot to her that they could be finally be reunited and cared for as a whole family.

For those involved in spiritual care, there is inspiration in recent writers who have sought to recover or reframe the ancient relationship between medicine and spirituality. The challenge for doctors of encompassing both curing and healing, or 'the two faces of medicine' (p.845), is described by Hutchinson, Hutchinson and Arnaert (2009); and the aspiration of reclaiming for modern, technological medicine

252 / CRITICAL CARE

a service-oriented model, in which 'spiritual or compassionate care involves serving the whole person' is documented by Puchalski (2001, p.352). Remen's stories (2006) disclose the 'hidden wholeness' of holding together curing *and* healing, along with both the medical *and* personal dimensions of people's lives. In one of them, she tells of a former gang member, whose young wife was dying of cancer, and a counselling session that she conducted with him, which was observed by a young psychiatrist. She describes how moving it was for the psychiatrist to hear the human and spiritual, as well as the medical and psychological dimensions of his history: how the man had discovered his own capacity for loving through the care he had given to his wife and to witness his hidden depths of tenderness. What emerges is not just the psychiatrist's reflection that 'we are all more than we seem', but her conclusion that 'actually, we are all more than we know. Wholeness is never lost, only forgotten' (Remen 2006, p.108).

The role of caring for the spirit involves seeking to understand some of the hidden meanings that people attribute to their experience. Reflecting on how spirituality is about the human struggle for ultimate purpose and meaning, or the underlying value of life, Stanworth (2004) tells the memorable story of the frail old lady, who refused to let her nurses clear away some dead flowers beside her bed, because 'as she watched the petals fall, "they help me to let go"' (p.2). It was as though they were helping her towards a new life, in the same way that Pooran's parents reframed their experience in terms of his helping his sister, Daiya, into this new life. Often we understand these things more by reflecting on our experience alongside families than by their disclosure of meaning, because their struggle is in caring for their child and family, day by day, hour by hour. I remember reflecting with a colleague on how my presence had worked out with a parent, whose children had been christened and attended church schools, but who had never seemed to wish to talk about faith. As we thought about this, it became apparent to us that since the child's illness had progressed so quickly, his parents were entirely caught up in keeping in step with him. From a faith perspective, they were treading the way of the cross, and worshipping him; for the time being, they had been wholly immersed in their journey, and they would only be able to talk or reflect on it at some point later on and further along the way.

There are times, though, when chaplaincy and spiritual care have a more explicit relation to the theme of wholeness, and an example of this was a creative art project to celebrate the 25th birthday of the hospice a few years ago. Two artist colleagues and I invited colleagues to reflect on something they enjoyed and valued here, first representing it creatively themselves through some artwork on a small canvas, and then enabling the children and families to follow suit. What was significant to me was how it affirmed the hospice as a whole community, because everyone was able to participate, while it also brought the meaning of our work into sharper focus. Children with profound impairments found help to decorate their canvases just as well as artistically gifted parents or highly qualified doctors, and their work is displayed together. Values such as hope and courage sat alongside fun, friendship, and having time to play and make memories, but the importance of things like a well-made cup of tea were not overlooked! While each canvas had a personal meaning, together they formed an image of the whole; and, as a whole, they speak powerfully to welcome people entering the hospice, for they reveal unequivocally the colour and light, as well as the shade and darkness, that characterise human experience here. Overall, they remind me of some words of the Canadian palliative care doctor, Balfour Mount, who said,

> My thoughts have been shaped by multiple personal brushes with death… (but) paradoxically, the message from these experiences has been about living, not dying. The psyche, it seems, has an intrinsic tendency toward healing, a will to wholeness, as it were. (Quoted in Gottlieb 2013, p.65)

A second example, which belongs more in the shade and darkness of experience at the hospice, reveals how hidden this wholeness can be for families. Another baby had come to our chilled bedroom, stillborn at 36 weeks in hospital, and unusually it fell to me to screw down the coffin lid in the presence of his parents. At this moment, I felt a profound sense of vulnerability and inadequacy, as though we were standing in the middle of an empty circle. It felt like an abyss of lost dreams; and as though the only 'wholeness' was the completeness of the sorrow that had engulfed this mother and father. It was only later, after some reflection, that I came to see how my presence, like that of my colleagues on similar occasions, might have made some difference. I realised how, unlike a hospital morgue, the room itself allows families to continue their relationship with their child even in death, and enables them to participate in the whole of their experience. Strange as it sounds, it seemed that I had been stood, not only in the heart of the circle, but also at the circumference. Being with them, standing by them and bearing witness to their experience, so that they were not alone, meant that they were also held and enfolded. It allowed them a measure of control as they sought some closure and completion: for not only had the baby's mother chosen during pregnancy to carry him as near as possible to term and also to come to the hospice, but with his father she had negotiated this ending in her own way and her own time.

Part two: Practices of faith and holiness

Contemplative practices, such as prayer and meditation, or mindfulness, are important for chaplaincy here, since being inwardly still and centred is essential for this work. The slow, faithful repetition of a prayer word, for example, is an ancient way of travelling beyond the grasping tendency of the mind; like a labyrinth, it takes us round and through the layers of the unconscious, and down into the mystery of love at the centre of our inner being. Freeman (2014) writes that these practices 'help us retain a sacramental and symbolic relationship to life', and that this 'connection with the living mystery' sustains our connection with our real selves and therefore with others. In my experience, a short, slow morning walk around the edge of the hospice garden, which incorporates a moment before an icon of the Madonna and child Jesus in our chapel, sustains this connection with an 'enduring melody' (Mayne 2013) that can be heard through the turmoil of experience. In this children's setting, it is interesting that the psalmist's words, 'be still and know that I am God' (Ps 46:10) and Eliot's lines (1980), 'at the still point of the turning world...at the still point, there the dance is' (p.191), are echoed by Mattie Stepanek (2001) when he says,

> I have a song, deep in my heart,
> And only I can hear it.
> If I close my eyes and sit very still,
> It is so easy to listen to my song. (p.3)

What is significant for families at a hospice, it seems to me, is that a chaplain is walking on this way, and can both represent and be familiar with this mysterious and holy journey of faith, hope and love, with all the twists and turns of a spiral stairway.

These contemplative practices can have tangible benefits in hospice and palliative care contexts, because the interior stillness and centring that they nurture help us to be more attentive and open to others. When I reflected on the second example in the chilled bedroom, it seemed that it was my attentive presence that had made it possible to be with the bereaved parents at both the centre and circumference of their experience. Reflecting on another occasion, when I had entered the room of a very sick young woman, whose mother was with her, I remember thinking how it had helped preserve a fundamental openness to whatever arose, when it would have been so easy to close things down by making assumptions about the significance of faith or prayer at that time. These qualities of attentiveness and openness are also important in integrating culture and spirituality into our end-of-life care. I remember how my colleagues asked the parents of a Muslim girl, whose death appeared close, but who seemed intent on staying in their bedroom with her, if they wanted to do some memory-making activities, or even take her into the garden for a while. In fact, we discovered that they were quite content to be in their room, to pray and prepare for death in solemn ways, which encircled her within their tradition, culture and faith; and, if anything, it was our own cultural assumptions about death that made us question their choice. Practices that nurture qualities of being and watching can help us become more conscious of our tendency towards activism, and better understand rituals that themselves involve watchfulness or vigil at the end of life.

Disciplines of watchfulness and silence, prayer and mindfulness can also help us to be with others in their pain, and so assist them on the way towards wholeness. A story that illustrates this connection was related to me by a colleague, John Foskett, and concerned the work of Romana Negri, an Italian child neuropsychiatrist, in a hospital's neo-natal intensive care unit. From her observations, she saw that the parents and nurses found watching the distress of the severely pre-term babies extremely difficult because of the painful feelings it stirred up, so that the nurses in particular would only approach the incubators when the machinery was signalling a problem. As she herself continued to watch the babies, though, she noticed that the nurses began to watch too, and comment on what they observed, such as particular characteristics or responses they were making; and this pattern was followed by the parents. Interpreting her attentive presence in terms of 'thought', Negri wrote:

> If somebody was able to think about the baby, all the others around were stimulated to do so. A circle of thought would begin, that enveloped the baby and included observer, doctors, nurses, and parents…when the child is thought about, he improves. (1997, p.2)

From the viewpoint of spiritual care, practices such as centring prayer include what Keating (2012) calls 'the unloading of the unconscious' (p.45) or the release of the emotional pain of early life, which is stored in our bodies. By enabling some of our own pain to be healed in this way, they also enable us to help in the healing of others' pain by our presence with them, and the circles of our thought and love and prayer.

Chaplaincy and spiritual care are also about creating the space in which others can be attentive, and this was the case with the creative art project commemorating our 25th anniversary. Contemplative practices focus on the recovery of stillness and inner attentiveness, often also enabling us to recover our vision and perspective. In a similar way, the project created a space in which our team could be still alongside the children and families and listen to them. Even when their words were barely discernible and their language was non-verbal, what Mattie Stepanek calls their 'heart songs' frequently emerged, and the resulting 'gallery' of canvases was like a collective heart song. It revealed not only a fresh and vibrant vision of the hospice, but, like the gesture of Jesus in placing a child in the middle of things, an unexpected face of love and holiness. The project was underpinned by a faith in the values of children and young people, and reminded us of some of their wholly remarkable lives. One young woman spelt out 'hope' as an acronym for 'hang on, pain ends'. It told us both about how she would live life fully in the weeks that remained, because her pain had become better controlled, and about the final end of pain at the time of her death. Part of her legacy, though, was to challenge and encourage us to continue to live out the hope that she had found in this place.

The contemplative practices described here can be interpreted in the Christian terms of 'The sacrament of the present moment' (De Caussade 1989) and the 'Practice of the presence of God' (Brother Lawrence 2005). In the example of the baby, who was stillborn at 36 weeks, it was only retrospectively that I perceived the more explicitly religious resonances of what took place, and the powerful connections with the Christian story. The baby's mother mentioned afterwards that she was glad that someone connected with the church had placed her son in the coffin and sealed it; and the feeling of my experience was captured by Rohr's words (2004): 'the authentic foundation of all true religion is the rediscovery of the defaced image of God inside of the human person, inside of this world, in what will always feel like the naked and empty now' (p.125). This occasion was religious in that we came together in some kind of common faith and reverence for this baby's life, as we brought some closure on it. Significantly, though, the coffin was a colourful one, and the images of stars and moon on it, which were reminiscent of a baby's nursery, lent normal and personal associations to it. This meant that sealing the coffin was transformative, and acquired sacramental and Eucharistic dimensions, since it broke open the possibility of a new vision of him, which was characterised less by physical death and more by the remembrance of normality and life.

Part three: Some aspects of healing

Paediatric palliative care is about healing, as we have seen, in that it helps children and their families find a way from suffering towards a sense of wholeness, irrespective of a cure for their disease. Liben *et al.* (2008) write that 'reducing physical pain and other distressing symptoms' creates a space for 'the possibility of healing' (p.858); and this was illustrated in comments made to me by Anne-Marie, who said of the absence of fear or anger in her daughter, Tina, at the end of her life, 'the important things of the spirit were intact and whole'. Healing depends on the twin focus of our presence with the child and family, and of our helping them to find some meaning in their experience. In this way, Negri (1997) brought healing to the intensive care unit by staying with the pain of the premature babies, in order to reveal its meaning for the nurses and parents around her. Her presence transformed their experience by enabling them to relinquish their grief at the babies' distress, and notice the responses they were making. There is a hidden wholeness waiting to be disclosed, and it is the new, alternative narrative, incorporating and not negating the existing view of things that makes this possible. For those involved in spiritual care, contemplative practices can be healing in a similar way, and enable us to promote such healing, because they foster a twin focus, and help to turn our attention from ourselves towards the life in which we participate. As Rohr (2013) says, 'You are participating in a Love that is being given to you. You are not creating this. You are just allowing it, trusting it for the pure gift that it is' (p.17).

Chaplaincy and spiritual care, of course, are as much about the spoken word as about our silent presence, and simple words of prayer or blessing can have a healing power at the frontiers of life and death. O'Donohue (2007) writes of our human need to honour these frontiers, and 'retrieve and reawaken our capacity for blessing', because on either side of them 'there is a different geography of thinking, feeling, and being' (pp.205–206), and a recent example illustrates this. As she was leaving the hospice with her family for the funeral of her daughter, and having said goodbye to her before she was placed in her coffin, a mother quite spontaneously asked me to say some words for her departure. It was as though she understood instinctively that her daughter was making a rite of passage, and that she was on the threshold of a new relationship with her, which she wanted to acknowledge, even though she did not need to hear the words herself. It is the connection with our deepest longings, which she intuited here, that makes these words of prayer or blessing healing, as O'Donohue (2007) observes:

> Regardless of how we configure the eternal, the human heart continues to dream of a state of wholeness, that place where everything comes together, where loss will be made good… To invoke a blessing is to call some of that wholeness upon a person now. (p.211)

Chaplains also need to be able to notice how healing is enacted in everyday activities, as much as in prepared rituals. In his poem, 'Clearances 3', Seamus Heaney (1990) tells how a boyhood memory of peeling potatoes with his mother, when everyone else was at Mass, returned to his mind just before her death:

> So while the parish priest at her bedside
> Went hammer and tongs at the prayers for the dying…
> I remembered her head bent towards my head
> Her breath in mine…
> Never closer the whole rest of our lives. (p.227)

He suggests that it is the memory of this ordinary, but intimate, time together that carries the healing and holiness, which the rituals of Mass and prayer were intended to convey. At the hospice, the significance of these times, with all the love and mystery they contain, is also recognised. When some small farm animals were visiting, a newborn lamb was brought to the room of a sick baby called Thomas, and his parents were surprised when it lay down alongside him in his cot, and they spent several minutes simply breathing peacefully together. It was a healing time for the family because this fresh experience transformed any feelings of merely waiting for death; and when the lamb was later named Thomas after their son, it gave them a powerful sense of his legacy and connection with the wider world of nature. Heaney was described as exalting 'everyday miracles' (Nobel Media 2014) such as this, and prayers, blessings or rituals need to point to the love and mysteries of healing within the everyday, as well as beyond it. As Remen (2006) says, 'Ritual doesn't make mystery happen. It helps us see and experience something which is already real. It does not create the sacred, it only describes what is there and has always been there, deeply hidden in the obvious' (p.284).

Although often extremely emotional, the funeral rites that chaplains conduct for children can surround families with care, and mobilise the power of the community for healing. Some parents once asked me to take part, because this continued the care of the hospice, where their daughter had had several stays. Preparing the funeral service together was empowering, when so many aspects of their daughter's care had been taken out of their hands. There was some recovery of a wholeness, which the illness had jeopardised, as they began to reintegrate memories of both her medical history and personal story; and after the intensive hospital treatments, when she could stay only with her parents, it was now possible for the whole family and friends, young and old, to come together to affirm their love for her. The image that we used for the service was of her brief life being like a pebble thrown into the water, where it ripples out in greater circles, because of the way she had touched many hearts over a short period. At the same time, though, we also thought of the presence of those people with us encircling her parents and sibling in their grief, and surrounding them with their love and healing hands.

Chaplaincy, then, is a focus for the spiritual care given by all of the team in a children's hospice, which is a community that heals by helping sick children and their families find ways towards some sense of wholeness. Inasmuch as the hospice offers the possibility that symptoms can be managed, emotions contained and trials borne, the image of the circle represents the way in which families can be held here as they make this most daunting journey. The canvases in our art project suggest this containment and connection, since each one is part of a larger whole; none stands alone, but all can be seen as belonging. The hospice also heals because it acknowledges the reality of death while sustaining the hope of life. Although wholeness will always seem elusive and hidden for families whose child is dying, our work is to hold out the possibility of healing by affirming their love, which transcends death. This touched me when two brothers called Ben and Josh were preparing for the ritual of our Christmas nativity procession. They carefully made three crowns for the three kings they would portray together with Tom, their sick brother. Sadly, though,

Tom was unable to wear it, as his condition worsened, and he died soon afterwards, but Ben and Josh placed it on top of his coffin for his funeral, where it stood as a potent symbol of their love.

Conclusion

We have seen how chaplaincy and spiritual care in a children's hospice can be understood in terms of holding for others the hope of a wholeness that is often hidden, and sometimes lost, in the struggle of living with and caring for very sick children. Merton's words are echoed by Jung's injunction (1964), 'Become what you have always been, namely, the wholeness we have lost in the midst of our civilised, conscious existence, a wholeness that we always were without knowing it' (para. 722). They also resonate with Rohr's assertion (2010) that 'there is a part of you that is Love itself, and that is what we must fall *into*. It is already there.' In order to extend to families the possibility of healing, we need both the centring practices that we have mentioned, and the encircling care and supervision of others. The beauty of this task is that it is reciprocal, and, as well as giving, we receive from colleagues and families alike. We also receive from inspirational children and young people, like Mattie, whose resilience is conveyed when he says, 'Sometimes my body wakes me up and says "Hey, you haven't had pain in a while. How about pain?" And sometimes I can't breathe, and that's hard to live with. But I still celebrate life and don't give up' (Stepanek 2002). What we do is for the common good, as our art project shows, but the first and final inspiration for chaplains in the Christian tradition is Jesus, whose words, 'inasmuch as you did it to the least of these, you did it to me' (Mt 25:45), reveal him as the source of wholeness hidden in our work.

REFERENCES

Albert, M.S., Steven, T. DeKosky, S. T., Dickson, D., Dubois, D., Feldman, H.H., Fox, N.C., Gamst, A., Holtzman, D.M., Jagust, W.J., Petersen, R.C., Snyder, P.J., Carrillo, M.C., Thies, B. and Phelps, C.H. (2011) 'The diagnosis of mild cognitive impairment due to Alzheimer's disease: Recommendations from the National Institute on Aging – Alzheimer's Association workgroups on diagnostic guidelines for Alzheimer's disease.' *Alzheimer's and Dementia: The Journal of the Alzheimer's Association 7,* 3, 270–279. Available at: www.alzheimersanddementia.com/article/S1552-5260%2811%2900104-X/abstract (accessed 25 February 2015).

Allmark, P. (2002) 'Death with dignity.' *Journal of Medical Ethics 28,* 255–257.

Alzheimer's Society (2008) 'Mild cognitive impairment (Fact Sheet 470).' Available at: www.alzheimers.org.uk/factsheets (accessed 25 February 2015).

Badham, P. (1996) 'A Theological Examination of the Case for Euthanasia.' In P. Badham and P. Ballard (eds) *Facing Death: An Interdisciplinary Approach.* Cardiff, UK: University of Wales Press.

Benson, J. and Thistlethwaite, J. (2008) *Mental Health across Cultures: A Practical Guide for Health Professionals.* Oxford, UK: Radcliffe Publishing Ltd.

Bloch, S. and Heyd, D. (2009) 'Suicide.' In S. Bloch and S. Green (eds) *Psychiatric Ethics* (fourth edition). Oxford, UK: Oxford University Press.

Brother Lawrence (2005) *The Practice of the Presence of God.* Philadelphia, PA: The Griffin and Rowland Press.

Charmaz, K. (2006) *Constructing Grounded Theory: A Practical Guide through Qualitative Analysis.* London: Sage.

Clayton, M. (2013) 'Contemplative chaplaincy: A view from a children's hospice.' *Practical Theology 6,* 1, 35–50.

Cobb, M. and Robshaw, V. (eds) (1998) *Spiritual Challenge of Health Care.* Harlow, UK: Churchill Livingstone.

Crawford, R. (1991) *Can We Ever Kill? An Ethical Enquiry.* London: Darton, Longman and Todd.

Crites, S. (1971) 'The narrative quality of experience.' *Journal of the American Academy of Religion 39,* 391–411.

Dalby, P. (2011) 'To Live and Do and Help – A Life That's Worthwhile: Reflections on the Spiritual Meaning of Generosity for People Living with Dementia.' In A. Jewell (ed.) *Spirituality and Personhood in Dementia.* London: Jessica Kingsley Publishers,.

De Caussade, J.-P. (1989) *The Sacrament of the Present Moment.* New York: Harper Collins.

Deveson, A. (2003) *Resilience.* Sydney: Allen & Unwin.

Dignitas (2004) 'Memorandum.' Select Committee on the Assisted Dying for the Terminally Ill Bill, House of Lords (2004). Available at: www.publications.parliament.uk/pa/ld200405/ldselect/ldasdy/86/5020307.htm (accessed 25 February 2015).

Durkheim, E. (1912/2008) *The Elementary Forms of Religious Life.* Oxford, UK: Oxford Paperbacks.

Eliot, T.S. (1980) *Collected Poems.* London: Faber and Faber.

Elkins, D.N., Hestorm, L.J., Hughes, L.L., Leaf, J.A. and Saunders, C. (1988) 'Towards a humanistic-phenomenological spirituality.' *Journal of Humanistic Psychology 28,* 4, 5–18.

Feldman, H., Scheltens, P., Scarpini, E., Hermann, N., Mesenbrink, P., Mancione, L., Tekin, S., Lane, R. and Ferris, S. (2004) 'Behavioral symptoms in mild cognitive impairment.' *Neurology* 62, 7, 1199–1201.

Fowler, J.W. (1981) *Stages of Faith: The Psychology of Human Development and the Quest for Meaning.* London. Harper & Row Publishers.

Frankl, V.E. (1984) *Man's Search for Meaning: An Introduction to Logotherapy.* New York: Simon & Schuster, Inc.

Freeman, L. (1999) *Practising Dying: The Work of Detachment* (Audio tape). London: Medio Media.

Freeman, L. (2014) *Lent Reflections Friday Week Four.* London: WCCM.

Garand, L., Dew, M.A., Eazor, L.R., DeKosky, S.T. and Reynolds, C.F. (2005) 'Caregiving burden and psychiatric morbidity in spouses of persons with mild cognitive impairment.' *International Journal of Geriatric Psychiatry 20,* 6, 512–522.

Gauthier, S., Reisberg, B., Zaudig, M., Peterson, R.C., Ritchie, K., Broich, K., Belleville, S., Brodaty, H., Bennett, D., Chertkow, H., Cummings, J., de Leon, M., Feldman, H., Ganguli, M., Hampel, H., Scheltens, P., Tierney, M.C., Whitehouse, P. and Winblad, B. (2006) 'Mild Cognitive Impairment.' *Lancet 367,* 9518, 1262–1270.

Gilbert, P. (2011) *Spirituality and Mental Health.* Brighton, UK: Pavillion.

Gottlieb, L. (2013) *Strengths-based Nursing Care: Health and Healing for Person and Family.* New York: Springer Publishing Company.

Hardy, D.W. (1996) *God's Ways with the World.* Edinburgh, UK: T and T Clark.

Hardy, D.W. (2001) *Finding the Church.* London: SCM Press.

Heaney, S. (1990) *New Selected Poems, 1966–1987.* London: Faber and Faber.

Hutchinson, T.A., Hutchinson, N. and Arnaert, A. (2009) 'Whole person care: Encompassing the two faces of medicine.' *Canadian Medical Association Journal 180,* 8, 845–846.

Johnston, W. (1995) *Mystical Theology.* London: Fount.

Jung, C.G. (1964) *Civilisation in Transition. Collected Works of C. G. Jung Volume 10.* London: Routledge and Kegan Paul.

Kaufman, Y., Anaki, D., Binns, M. and Freedman, M. (2007) 'Cognitive decline in Alzheimer disease: Impact of spirituality, religiosity, and QOL.' *Neurology 68,* 18, 1509–1514.

Keating, T. (2012) *Intimacy with God: An Introduction to Centering Prayer.* New York: Crossroad Publishing Company.

Kennedy, J., Stirling, I., McKenzie, D. and Wallace, D. (2013) 'Developing innovation in spiritual care education: Research in primary health and social care.' Edinburgh: NHS NES. Available at: www.animateconsulting.org.uk/wp-content/uploads/2013/09/Chaplaincy-Report_23.01.13.pdf (accessed 25 February 2015).

Kitwood, T. (1997) *Dementia Reconsidered: The Person Comes First.* Buckingham, UK: Open University Press.

Küng, H. (1995) *A Dignified Dying.* London: SCM Press Ltd.

Lash, N. (1996) *The Beginning and End of Religion.* Cambridge, UK: Cambridge University Press.

Laverty, S.M. 'Hermeneutic Phenomenology and Phenomenology: A Comparison of Historical and Methodological Considerations.' *International Journal of Qualitative Methods 2,* 3, September 2003.

Liben, S., Papadatou, D. and Wolfe, J. (2008) 'Paediatric palliative care: Challenges and emerging ideas.' *The Lancet 371,* 9615, 852–864.

Licqurish, S. and Seibold, C. (2011) 'Applying a contemporary Grounded Theory methodology.' *Nurse Researcher 18,* 4, 11–16.

Lloyd, M. (2006) 'Resilience promotion – its role in clinical medicine.' *Australian Family Physician 35,* 1–2, 63–64.

Lloyd, M. (2011) 'Resilience Promotion and its Relevance to the Personhood Needs of People with dementia and Other Brain Damage.' In A. Jewell (ed.) *Spirituality and Personhood in Dementia.* London: Jessica Kingsley Publishers.

Lu, Y.-F., Haase, E. and Farran, C. (2007) 'Perspectives of persons with mild cognitive impairment: Sense of being able.' *Alzheimer's Care Quarterly 8,* 1, 75–86.

Macauley, R. and Hylton Rushton, C. (2012) 'Spirituality and Meaning for Children, Families and Clinicians.' In A. Goldman, R. Hain, and S. Liben (eds) *Oxford Textbook of Palliative Care for Children* (second edition). Oxford, UK: Oxford University Press.

MacKinlay, E. (2006) *Spiritual Growth and Care in the Fourth Age of Life.* London: Jessica Kingsley Publishers.

McDonnell, T.P. (ed.) (1989) *A Thomas Merton Reader.* London: Lamp Press.

McSherry, W. (2006) *Making Sense of Spirituality in Nursing and Health Care Practice: An Interactive Approach* (second edition). London: Jessica Kingsley Publishers.

Martin, D. (1980) *The Breaking of the Image.* Oxford, UK: Basil Blackwell.

Martinez, R. (2009) 'Narrative Ethics.' In S. Bloch and S. Green (eds) *Psychiatric Ethics* (fourth edition). Oxford, UK: Oxford University Press.

Mayne, M. (2013) *The Enduring Melody.* London: Darton, Longman and Todd.

Mental Capacity Act (2005) 'Mental Capacity Act.' London: The Stationery Office. Available at: www.legislation.gov.uk/ukpga/2005/9/pdfs/ukpga_20050009_en.pdf (accessed 25 February 2015).

Mental Health Act (1983) 'Mental Health Act.' London: The Stationery Office. Available at: www.legislation.gov.uk/ukpga/1983/20/pdfs/ukpga_19830020_en.pdf (accessed 25 February 2015).

Naudts, K., Ducatelle, C., Kovacs, J., Laurens, K., Van Den Eynde, F. and Van Heeringen, C. (2006) 'Euthanasia: The role of the psychiatrist.' *British Journal of Psychiatry 188,* 405–409.

Negri, R. (1997) 'The newborn in the Department of Neonatal Intensive Care Unit (NICU): A neuropsychological model of prevention.' Unpublished paper, University of Milan.

Newell, T. (2002) 'Restorative Justice: An Expression of Spirituality Within Criminal Justice.' In C. Jones and P.H. Sedgwick (eds) *The Future of Criminal Justice: Resettlement, Chaplaincy and Community.* London: SPCK.

Nobel Media (2014) 'The Nobel Prize in Literature 1995.' Available at: www.nobelprize.org/nobel_prizes/literature/laureates/1995/ (accessed 25 February 2015).

O'Donohue, J. (2007) *Benedictus: A Book of Blessings.* London: Bantam Press.

Ochs, P. (2011) *Another Reformation: Postliberal Christianity and the Jews.* Grand Rapids, MI: Baker Academic.

Puchalski, C. (2001) 'The role of spirituality in health care.' *Proceedings of Baylor University Medical Center 14,* 4, 352–357.

Puchalski, C. (2006) *A Time for Listening and Caring: Spirituality and the Care of the Chronically Ill and Dying.* Oxford, UK: Oxford University Press.

Royal College of Nursing (2008) 'The RCN's definition of dignity.' Royal College of Nursing. Available at: www.rcn.org.uk/development/practice/dignity/rcns_definition_of_dignity (accessed 25 February 2015).

Rees, E. (2012) 'Ministering to those with Alzheimer's Disease and Related Disorders (ADRD).' Unpublished MTh essay, Cardiff University.

Remen, R. (2006) *Kitchen Table Wisdom: Stories that Heal.* New York: Riverhead Books.

Reynolds, D. (2013) *The Long Shadow.* London: Simon and Schuster.

Ritchie, K., Artero, S. and Touchon, J. (2001) 'Classification criteria for mild cognitive impairment: A population-based validation study.' *Neurology 56,* 37–42. Available at: www.neurology.org/content/56/1/37.full.pdf+html (accessed 25 February 2015).

Rohr, R. (2004) *Soul Brothers: Men in the Bible Speak to Men Today.* New York: Orbis Books.

Rohr, R. (2010) *The Art of Letting Go: Living the Wisdom of St Francis* (CD/audio book). Boulder, CO: Sounds True.

Rohr, R. (2011) *Falling Upward: A Spirituality for the Two Halves of Life.* London: SPCK.

Rohr, R. (2013) *Yes, and?* Cincinnati, OH: Franciscan Media.

Ruffing, J.K. (2011) *To Tell the Sacred Tale: Spiritual Direction and Narrative.* New York: Paulist Press.

Shamy, E. (2003) *A Guide to the Spiritual Dimension of Care for People with Alzheimer's Disease and Related Dementia: More than Body, Brain and Breath.* London: Jessica Kingsley Publishers.

Stanworth, R. (2004) *Recognising Spiritual Needs in People who are Dying.* Oxford, UK: Oxford University Press.

Stepanek, M.J.T. (2001) *Journey through Heartsongs.* New York: Hyperion.

Stepanek, M.J.T. (2002) 'Poet Mattie Stepanek helps "Jerry's kids".' Available at: http://
    usatoday30.usatoday.com/news/health/spotlighthealth/2002-08-30-mattie_x.htm
    (accessed 25 February 2015).

Swift, C. (2009) *Hospital Chaplaincy in the Twenty-first Century: The Crisis of Spiritual Care on the NHS.*
    Aldershot, UK: Ashgate.

Swinton, J. (2001) *Spirituality and Mental Health Care: Rediscovering a 'Forgotten' Dimension.* London:
    Jessica Kingsley Publishers.

Swinton, J. (2008) 'Remembering the Person: Theological Reflections on God, Personhood and
    Dementia.' In E. MacKinlay (ed.) *Ageing, Disability and Spirituality: Addressing the Challenge of
    Disability in Later Life.* London: Jessica Kingsley Publishers.

Swinton, J. and Mowat, H. (2006) *Practical Theology and Qualitative Research.* London: SCM Press.

Swinton, J. and Payne, R. (eds) (2009) *Living Well and Dying Faithfully.* Grand Rapids, MI: William
    B. Eerdmans Publishing.

Taylor, C. (2007) *A Secular Age.* Cambridge, MA: Belknap Press of Harvard University Press.

Tutu, D. (1999) *No Future without Forgiveness: A Personal Overview of South Africa's Truth and
    Reconciliation Committee.* London: Rider Books.

Vanier, J. (1999) *Becoming Human.* New York: Paulist Press.

White, G. (2006) *Talking about Spirituality in Health Care Practice: A Resource for the Multi-professional
    Health Care Team.* London: Jessica Kingsley Publishers.

WHO (2014) 'WHO Definition of Palliative Care.' Available at: www.who.int/cancer/palliative/
    definition/en (accessed 25 February 2015).

Williams, R. (2000) *Christ on Trial.* London: Harper Collins.

CONTRIBUTORS

Rev Dr Jonathan Pye

Jonathan Pye is a Methodist Minister, Honorary Research Fellow at the Centre for Ethics in Medicine/Research Associate in the School of Community and Social Medicine, University of Bristol. He is a Tutor on the MTh in Chaplaincy Studies at the University of Cardiff. An experienced former hospital chaplain, he is the author of *Dementia: the Challenge to Care* (Brisbane: Blue Nursing) and numerous articles. He is Healing Advisor to the Cumbria Methodist District and the Anglican Diocese of Carlisle.

Rev Hamish Ferguson-Stuart

Hamish Ferguson-Stuart is an Anglican priest and a graduate of the MTh in Chaplaincy at Cardiff University. He is currently a member of the chaplaincy team, Rotherham NHS Foundation Trust, South Yorkshire.

Rev Stephen Flatt

Stephen Flatt is a Registered Nurse and Anglican priest. He currently works as the Hospital Site Matron at Newham University Hospital, part of Barts Health NHS Trust, as well as being a self-supporting priest in the clergy team at the Annunciation, Marble Arch. He is a graduate of MTh in Chaplaincy from Cardiff University and is currently researching a doctorate exploring the role of the multi-disciplinary healthcare team in delivering spiritual care in the acute healthcare setting.

Rev Anne McCormick

Anne McCormick has been an Anglican priest for 20 years. She is currently a chaplain in an acute hospital setting in Lincolnshire and formerly served as a mental health chaplain. Her first degree was in Biblical studies at Sheffield University and she is a graduate of the MTh in Chaplaincy at

266 / CRITICAL CARE

Cardiff University. She holds a PGCE in teaching RE and History from Hull and has taught Old Testament courses for ministry training candidates, both lay and ordained within the Diocese of Lincoln.

Rev Dr Andrew Todd

Andrew Todd is an Anglican priest, a practical theologian and ethnographer and manages the Cardiff Centre for Chaplaincy Studies where he also directs its research programme. Andrew has been involved in research into chaplaincy in different settings, including prisons, the Armed Forces and healthcare. He is the editor of *Military Chaplaincy in Contention: Chaplains, Churches, and the Morality of Conflict* (Ashgate Press). He is also Senior Associate of the Cambridge Theological Federation.

Dr Layla Welford

Layla Welford graduated from Cardiff University in law in 2007 and then completed a PhD at Cardiff University in 2010 on Spiritual Healthcare and Public Policy, focussing on the impact of legislation and social policy on the provision of healthcare chaplaincy in England and Wales. She is now a research associate of the Cardiff University Centre for Law and Religion and currently serving in full-time ministry with Mosaic, Los Angeles.

Mirabai Galashan

Mirabai Galashan is a Healthcare Chaplain, writer and holistic therapist. She is a graduate of the MTh in Chaplaincy at Cardiff University. She pioneered the role of Chaplain to the palliative care team of the Children's Hospital of Philadelphia and has extensive experience in hospital and hospice chaplaincy. Her post-graduate research inspired her to lead a task force for the Association of Professional Chaplains to review inclusivity and diversity in the board certification process.

Rev Debbie Hodge

Rev Debbie Hodge is a minister of the United Reformed Church. Prior to ordination she was Principal Lecturer in Nursing Studies at Hertfordshire University. Her current roles include; Secretary for Health Care Chaplaincy for the Free Churches Group; Chief Officer of the Health Care Chaplaincy Faith and Belief Group and is a member of the Editorial

Board of 'Health and Social Care Chaplaincy'. Debbie is currently co-researching the priorities for End of Life Care.

Rev Dr Steve Nolan

Steve Nolan has been chaplain at Princess Alice Hospice, Esher, UK since 2004. He holds a PhD from the University of Manchester and is dual qualified as a BACP accredited counsellor/psychotherapist. Previous publications include, *Spiritual Care at the End of Life: The Chaplain as a 'Hopeful Presence'* (Jessica Kingsley Publishers, 2012) and (co-edited with George Fitchett) *Spiritual Care in Practice: Case Studies in Healthcare Chaplaincy* (Jessica Kingsley Publishers, 2015).

Rev Julian Raffay

Julian works as Specialist Chaplain (Research, Education and Development) at Mersey Care NHS Trust. He is currently researching how co-production principles could improve mental health spiritual and pastoral care (chaplaincy) services in partnership with the Cardiff Centre for Chaplaincy Studies. He was previously at Sheffield Health and Social Care NHS Foundation Trust where he worked as Chaplaincy Team Leader and has published a number of articles on spiritual care.

Rev Canon Karen MacKinnon

Karen MacKinnon is the professional officer (South Central) for The College of Healthcare Chaplains. She was the youngest of the first 32 women ordained priest in the Church of England. She left parish ministry in 2000 wanting to specialise in healthcare chaplaincy and is the Head of the Spiritual Care Service at University Hospital Southampton NHS Foundation Trust where she launched the Trust's first Spiritual Care Policy in 2010. She is a graduate of the MTh in Chaplaincy from Cardiff University. She is Bishop's Advisor for Health Care Chaplaincy in Winchester Diocese.

Rev Rodney Baxendale

Rodney Baxendale originally trained as a Drama teacher, has served twice in the Royal Navy: as an Instructor Officer, and then as a Chaplain, serving in many ships and establishments, finally in RFA ARGUS, the navy's hospital ship. After retirement, he has been Lead Chaplain at Derriford Hospital, and since his second retirement now works part-time there and in St Luke's Hospice in Plymouth.

Rev Dr Peter Sedgwick

Peter Sedgwick is an Anglican priest, a Life Fellow at the Center for Theological Inquiry at Princeton University, New Jersey, USA, Honorary Lecturer at the School of History, Archaeology and Religion at Cardiff University, and was the Principal of St Michael's College, Llandaff. He is the author of several theological books and numerous articles.

Rev Charles Thody

Charles Thody is an Anglican Priest and Senior Healthcare Chaplain, currently working as Lead Chaplain to a large general healthcare Trust. He is a graduate of the MTh in Chaplaincy at Cardiff University. Much of his chaplaincy career has been in mental health, with a particular interest in forensic psychiatry and personality disorders, having been Lead Chaplain at Rampton High Secure Hospital.

Rev Richard Wharton

Richard Wharton an Anglican priest and the Team Leader of a multi-faith Chaplaincy at University Hospital Birmingham. He is a graduate of the MTh in Chaplaincy at Cardiff University, where he explored creative expressions of spiritual care amongst those living with cognitive impairment. He is also interested in how the Christian contemplative traditions can inform spiritual care in a culturally diverse setting.

Rev Mark Clayton

Mark Clayton is a chaplain at Martin House children's hospice, which is located between Leeds and York in West Yorkshire. The hospice was the second in this country, and indeed the world, when it opened in 1987. As a chaplain, he is interested in the connection between prayer and care; and how the Christian contemplative tradition can inform contemporary pastoral and spiritual care.

SUBJECT INDEX

AUTHOR INDEX